SMOKING AND REPRODUCTIVE HEALTH

Edited by

Michael J. Rosenberg, M.D., M.P.H.

PSG Publishing Company, Inc.
Littleton, Massachusetts

Library of Congress Cataloging-in-Publication Data

Smoking and reproductive health.

Based on the International Conference on Smoking and Reproductive Health, held on Oct. 16-18, 1985, in San Francisco, Calif.
Includes index.
1. Smoking--Physiological effect--Congresses. 2. Tobacco--Toxicology--Congresses. 3. Fetus--Effect of drugs on--Congresses. 4. Generative organs--Effect of drugs on--Congresses. 5. Smoking--Government policy--Congresses. I. Rosenberg, Michael J. II. International Conference on Smoking and Reproductive Health (1985 : San Francisco, Calif.) [DNLM: 1. Infertility--etiology--congresses. 2. Neoplasms--etiology--congresses. 3. Pregnancy Complications--etiology--congresses. 4. Public Policy--congresses. 5. Reproduction--drug effects--congresses. 6. Smoking--in pregnancy--congresses. WQ 240 S666 1985]
RG627.6.T6S66 1986 618.2 86-25604
ISBN 0-88416-549-3

Printed in United States of America.

International Standard Book Number: 0-88416-549-3

Library of Congress Catalog Card Number: 86-25604

Last digit is print number: 9 8 7 6 5 4 3 2 1

Contributors

David Acker, M.D.
Associate Chief, Department of Obstetrics and Gynecology
Beth Israel Hospital
Boston, Massachusetts

Elba Beatriz Aquirre, M.D.
Assistant Professor, Obstetrics
Hospital General de Agudos
Capital Federal, Argentina

Sherrie S. Aitken, D.P.A.
Vice President
CSR, Incorporated
Washington, D.C.

Husain A. Al-Mumen, M.D., M.P.H.
Vice President
Kuwait Smoking and Cancer Prevention Society
Safat, Kuwait

M.A. Arabi, M.D., M.R.C.P.
Consultant Physician
Omdurman Hospital
Ministry of Health
Khartoum, Sudan

Elaine Bratic Arkin
Deputy Director, Office of Public Affairs
U.S. Public Health Service
Washington, D.C.

Ramon Aznar
Head, Contraception Methodology
Centro de Investigacion
Sobre Fertilidad y Eterlidad
Mexico, City, Mexico

Mohamed Bailey
Graduate Fellow
College of Social Sciences
Center for the Study of Population
Florida State University
Tallahassee, Florida

John A. Baron, M.D,
Assistant Professor of Internal Medicine
Dartmouth Medical School
Dartmouth, New Hampshire

Heinz W. Berendes, M.D., M.H.S.
Director, Epidemiology and Biometry Research Program
National Institute of Child Health and Development
Bethesda, Maryland

Reinhold Bergstrom, Ph.D.
Associate Director, Department of Statistics
University of Uppsala
Uppsala, Sweden

Stuart Berman
Medical Epidemiologist, Division of Sexually Transmitted Diseases
Center for Prevention Services
Centers for Disease Control
Atlanta, Georgia

Edward N. Brandt, Jr., M.D., Ph.D.
Chancellor
University of Maryland at Baltimore
Baltimore, Maryland

Dee Burton, Ph.D.
Director of Adult Education
Health Behavior Research Institute
University of California
Pasedena, California

Oona Campbell, Sc.M.
Doctoral Candidate
Johns Hopkins University
Baltimore, Maryland

Graham A. Colditz, M.B.B.S., M.P.H.
Instructor in Medicine, Department of Medicine
Harvard Medical School and Brigham and Women's Hospital
Department of Epidemiology
Harvard School of Public Health
Brookline, Massachusetts

L. Collins-Burris
Smoking Counsellor, Department of Obstetrics and Gynecology
University Health Center
Office of Health Promotion Research
University of Vermont
Burlington, Vermont

Janet R. Daling, Ph.D.
Associate Professor, Department of Epidemiology
University of Washington
Seattle, Washington

Thomas E. Delea, B.A.
Research Assistant
Policy Analysis Inc.
Brookline, Massachusetts

Jacques de Mouzon, M.D.
Research Officer
Institut National de la Sante et de la Recherche Medicale
Paris, France

Issaac W. Eberstein, Ph.D.
Research Associate and Associate Professor
College of Social Sciences
Center for the Study of Population
Florida State University
Tallahassee, Florida

Anders Ericson, M.Sc
Director
National Board of Health and Welfare
Stockholm, Sweden

Virginia L. Ernster, Ph.D.
Associate Professor of Epidemiology, Department of Epidemiology and International Health
School of Medicine
University of California
San Francisco, California

Trena Ezzati, M.S.
Survey Statistician
National Center for Health Statistics
Hyattsville, Maryland

B.S. Flynn, Sc.D.
Associate Director
Office of Health Promotion Research
Division of Health Sciences
College of Medicine
University of Vermont
Burlington, Vermont

Norma Lynn Fox, Ph.D.
Assistant Professor, Department of Epidemiology and Preventive Medicine
School of Medicine
University of Maryland
Baltimore, Maryland

Adele L. Franks, M.D.
Medical Epidemiologist
Epidemiologic Studies Branch
Division for Reproductive Health
Center for Health Promotion and Education
Centers for Disease Control
Atlanta, Georgia

Thomas J. Glynn, Ph.D.
Program Director for Smoking Research
National Cancer Institute
Preventive Research Branch
Division of Clinical Research
Bethesda, Maryland

Ronald Gray, M.B., B.S.
Professor, Department of Population Dynamics
School of Hygiene and Public Health
Johns Hopkins University
Baltimore, Maryland

E. Robert Greenberg, M.D.
Associate Professor, Department of Community and Family Medicine
Dartmouth Medical School
Dartmouth, New Hampshire

Gary S. Grubb, M.D., M.P.H.
Medical Epidemiologist
Division of Reproductive Epidemiology
Family Health International
Research Triangle Park, North Carolina

Susan Harlap, M.B.B.S.
Associate Professor of Epidemiology and Public Health, Department of Medical Ecology
Hadassah Medical School
Hebrew University
Jerusalem, Israel

J. Richard Hebel, Ph.D.
Professor, Department of Epidemiology and Preventive Medicine
School of Medicine
University of Maryland
Baltimore, Maryland

Lothar Heinemann
Professor, Department of Epidemiology and Preventive Medicine
Academie der Wissenschaften der DDR
Forshungszentrum fur Molekularbiologie und Medizin
Berlin, Germany

Jerry Hendershot, Ph.D.
Chief, Illness and Disability Statistics Branch
Division of Health Interview Statistics
National Center for Health
Hyattsville, Maryland

James E. Higgins, Ph.D.
Senior Biostatistician
Biostatistics and Quality Assurance
Family Health International
Research Triangle Park, North Carolina

Howard J. Hoffman, M.D.
Chief, Biometry Branch
National Institute of Child Health and Development
Bethesda, Maryland

Carol J.R. Hogue, Ph.D.
Chief, Pregnancy Epidemiology Branch
Division of Reproductive Health
Center for Health Promotion and Education
Centers for Disease Control
Atlanta, Georgia

Susan Holck, M.D.
Medical Officer
Special Programme of Research, Development, and Research Training in Human Reproduction
World Health Organization
Geneva, Switzerland

Thomas T. Kane, Ph.D.
Research Associate
Program Evaluation Division
Family Health International
Research Triangle Park, North Carolina

Kenneth G. Keppel, Ph.D.
Statistician
Division of Vital Statistics
National Center for Health Statistics
Hyattsville, Maryland

Ronald M. Krauss, M.D.
Senior Staff Statistician
University of California
Berkeley, California

Robert LaForge, Ph.D.
Associate
Alcohol Epidemiologic Data System
Washington, D.C.

Garland Land, M.P.H.
Deputy Director
Health Resources
Missouri Department of Health
Jefferson City, Missouri

Peter M. Layde, M.D.
Director, Division of Chronic Disease Control
Center for Environmental Health
Centers for Disease Control
Atlanta, Georgia

S. LePage, R.N.
Smoking Counsellor, Department of Obstetrics and Gynecology
University Health Center
Office of Health Promotion Research
Division of Health Sciences
Burlington, Vermont

Samuel M. Lesko, M.D.
Senior Epidemiologist
Drug Epidemiology Unit
Brookline, Massachusetts

Greg Lieberknecht, M.S.
Computer Programmer
Kaiser Permanente Medical Care Program
Walnut Creek, California

Henry Malin
Social Scientist
National Institute on Alcohol Abuse and Alcoholism
Rockville, Maryland

Michael Marmot
Chairman, Department of Community Medicine
University College, London, and
The Middlesex Hospital Medical School
London, England

Roberto Masironi, M.D.
Coordinator
WHO Programme on Smoking and Health
Geneva, Switzerland

Donald R. Mattison, M.D.
Associate Professor, Department of Obstetrics and Gynecology
Director of Reproductive Pharmacology and Toxicology
University of Arkansas for Medical Sciences
Little Rock, Arkansas

B.V. McPherson, M.S.
Biostatistician
College of Medicine
Biometry Facility
University of Vermont
Burlington, Vermont

P. Mead, M.D.
Clinical Professor, Department of Obstetrics and Gynecology
College of Medicine
University of Vermont
Burlington, Vermont

Ernesto Medina, M.D., M.P.H.
Director, School of Public Health
University of Chile
Santiago, Chile

Olav Meirik, M.D., Ph.D.
Associate Professor, Department of Social Medicine
University Hospital
Uppsala, Sweden

Karen Monaco, M.S.
Manager, Smoking or Health
American Lung Association
New York, New York

Donald E. Moore, M.D.
Associate Professor, Department of Obstetrics and Gynecology
University of Washington
Seattle, Washington

Abigail J. Moss
Health Statistician
Division of Health Interview Statistics
National Center for Health
Hyattsville, Maryland

Howard Ory, M.D.
Medical Epidemiologist
Division of Information Resources Management Office
Centers for Disease Control
Atlanta, Georgia

Gerry Oster, Ph.D.
Vice President
Policy Analysis, Inc.
Brookline, Massachusetts

Mary D. Overpeck, M.P.H.
Health Statistician
Biometry Branch
National Institute of Child Health and Development
Bethesda, Maryland

Jeffrey A. Perlman, M.D., M.S.C.
Chief, Contraceptive Evaluation Branch
National Institute of Child Health and Development
Bethesda, Maryland

John Pinney
Executive Director
Institute for the Study of Smoking Behavior and Policy
Kennedy School of Government
Cambridge, Massachusetts

Paul Placek, Ph.D.
Social Scientist
National Center for Health Statistics
Hyattsville, Maryland

J.O.M. Pobee, M.B., F.R.C.P.
Chief, Department of Internal Medicine
Professor and Chairman, Department of Medicine and Therapeutics
University of Ghana Medical School
Accra, Ghana

Reimert Ravenholt, M.D., M.P.H.
Director, World Health Surveys, Inc.
Bethesda, Maryland

Rose Ray, Ph.D.
Statistical Consultant
University of California
Berkeley, California

Mario Rigatto, M.D.
President
Latin American Coordinating Committee for Smoking Control
Professor of Medicine
Federal University of Rio Grande do Sul
Porto Alegre, Brazil

Lynn Rosenberg, Sc.D.
Assistant Director
Boston University School of Medicine
Drug Epidemiology Unit
Brookline, Massachusetts

Michael Rosenberg, M.D., M.P.H.
Director, Reproductive Epidemiology Division
Family Health International
Research Triangle Park, North Carolina
Adjunct Assistant Professor of Epidemiology
University of North Carolina

George L. Rubin, M.B.B.S.
Chief, Epidemiologic Studies Branch
Center for Health Promotion
Division of Reproductive Health
Centers for Disease Control
Atlanta, Georgia

Ronnette Russell-Briefel, Ph.D.
Epidemiologist
National Center for Health Statistics
Hyattsville, Maryland

Benjamin P. Sachs, M.D., D.P.H.
Director, Division of Maternal and Fetal Medicine
Beth Israel Hospital
Assistant Professor of Obstetrics and Gynecology
Harvard Medical School
Harvard School of Public Health
Boston, Massachusetts

William Sappenfield, M.D.
Medical Epidemiologist
Pregnancy Epidemiology Branch
Division of Reproductive Health
Center for Health Promotion and Education
Centers for Disease Control
Atlanta, Georgia

Daniel Schwartz, Ph.D.
Professor
Institut National de la Sante et de la Recherche Medicale
Paris, France

Roger H. Secker-Walker, M.B., F.R.C.P.
Professor of Medicine
Director of Health Promotion Research
Division of Health Sciences
Burlington, Vermont

Mary Sexton, Ph.D., P.P.H.
Professor, Department of Epidemiology and Preventive Medicine
School of Medicine
University of Maryland
Baltimore, Maryland

M. Shipley
Statistician
London School of Hygiene and Tropical Medicine
London, England

Donald R. Shopland
Acting Director
Office on Smoking and Health
Public Health Service
U.S. Department of Health and Human Services
Rockville, Maryland

Jason B. Smith, M.P.H.
Project Coordinator
Center for Development and Population Activities
Washington, D.C.

L.J. Solomon, Ph.D.
Clinical Assistant Professor
College of Medicine
University of Vermont
Burlington, Vermont

Leon R. Spadoni, M.D.
Professor, Department of Obstetrics and Gynecology
University of Washington
Seattle, Washington

Daniel Spiegler
Social Scientist
National Institute on Alcohol Abuse and Alcoholism
Division of Biometry and Epidemiology
Rockville, Maryland

Alfred Spira, M.D., Ph.D.
Associate Professeur
Institut National de la Sante et de la Recherche Medicale
Paris, France

Bruce V. Stadel, M.D.
Medical Officer
National Institute of Child Health and Development
Washington, D.C.

Joseph W. Stockbauer, M.A.
Presearch Analyst III
Health Resources
Missouri Department of Health
Jefferson City, Missouri

Nancy E. Stroup, Ph.D.
Epidemiologist
Center for Environmental Health
Division of Chronic Disease Control
Centers for Disease Control
Atlanta, Georgia

Shanna Swan, Ph.D.
Chief, Methodology and Analysis Unit
Department of Health Services
Epidemiological Studies and Surveillance Section
Berkeley, California

Selma M. Taffel, B.B.A.
Statistician
Division of Vital Statistics
National Center for Health Statistics
Hyattsville, Maryland

Peter J. Thomford, Ph.D.
Instructor, Department of Obstetrics and Gynecology
University of Arkansas for Medical Sciences
Little Rock, Arkansas

Lynda F. Voigt, M.S.
Research Associate
Fred Hutchinson Cancer Research Center
Seattle, Washington

Rebecca Wang
Lecturer, Department of Medicine
University of Hong Kong
Queen Mary Hospital
Hong Kong

Diana Chapman Walsh, Ph.D.
Associate Director
Health Policy Institute
Assistant Professor of Public Health
Boston University
Boston, Massachusetts

Linda A. Webster, M.P.H.
Statistician
Center for Health Promotion and Education
Division of Reproductive Health
Centers for Disease Control
Atlanta, Georgia

Noel S. Weiss, M.D., D.P.H.
Professor, Department of Epidemiology
University of Washington
Seattle, Washington

Robert H. Weller, Ph.D.
Professor
College of Social Sciences
Center for the Study of Population
Florida State University
Tallahassee, Florida

Susan Wilner, Sc.D., M.P.H.
Health Policy Scholar
Institute for Health Policy Studies
Medical Center
University of California
San Francisco, California

Phyllis A. Wingo, M.P.H.
Statistician
Center for Health Promotion and Education
Division of Reproductive Health
Centers for Disease Control
Atlanta, Georgia

Contents

Preface

We recently experienced one of the worst years in aviation history. The concern that surrounds the safety issue is reflected by stories splashed across every major newspaper. This concern is understandable and justified, but in terms of public health and preventable deaths, consider that each year approximately 350,000 people die because they used tobacco products. This is the equivalent of three 747 crashes per day, year after year.

C. Everett Koop, the US Surgeon General, labels cigarette smoking as the "chief, single avoidable cause of death in our society and the most important public health issue of our time." Yet despite decades of research which has established tobacco as a health hazard, a chasm exists between this knowledge and our societal inability to control tobacco use.

Smoking prevalence has increased markedly in the United States over the last 50 years. The increased consumption of cigarettes has not been limited to the United States, or even the developed nations. Studies reflect high and increasing cigarette consumption throughout the world, encouraged by advertising which portrays smoking as being sophisticated, glamorous, and virile. In most countries, more than 20% of young men smoke regularly. Europe and some Latin American countries—Argentina, Chile, and Uruguay—have similar prevalence rates of smoking among 15-year-old girls and boys. In Senegal, 70% of schoolboys smoke. While smoking in young women is less common, generally ranging between 0% and 33%, a troublesome increase has occurred among this group. In the United States, for example, there has been a 50% increase in the proportion of girls aged 12 to 18 years who smoke, in contrast to a 30% decrease among boys of the same age. Globally, this increase is doubly disturbing, since we can well estimate the resulting illness and death which will occur in the future as a consequence.

I stress the word illness. This book deals not so much with the mortality of 1000 747's crashes every year, but rather explores some of the newly recognized and more subtle effects of smoking. Tobacco smoking exposes every tissue and cell in a smoker's body to circulating mutagens. It is not surprising, then, that an increasing body of literature indicates with mounting certainty that smoking adversely affects the reproductive system, particularly those portions with rapid cellular growth such as the gonads and the developing embryo. As compared with the established carcinogenic effects of smoking, the reproductive consequences affect a younger group in more subtle ways. Adverse reproductive events such as increased difficulty in becoming pregnant, or higher rates of fetal loss, tend to be more private matters than cancer. These events of early adult life tend to be felt long before the other health effects of smoking and so are of great concern to persons from the developing world.

Over the last 30 years, and particularly over the past decade, a trickle of journal articles has become a steady stream revealing a variety of reproductive problems associated with smoking. These problems include contraindication to use of certain contraceptives, impaired conception and fetal development, and problems with delivery, infant development, and cancers of the reproductive system. Summarizing this recent knowledge, along with previous work, is the first objective of this book.

The second emphasis is a critical summary of smoking prevention and cessation efforts. Approximately 20% of pregnant women stop smoking when they become pregnant, but the remainder pose questions about the most effective intervention strategies. What is clear is that health care providers are most effective, but the type and content of antismoking messages, and specific strategies tailored to certain groups of men as well women, need to be clarified.

The final goal is to provide a forum for presenting the interests of an increasingly vocal group of nonsmokers in a society which also emphasizes the rights of smokers. As the meeting on which this book is based took place in San Francisco, a city which forbids smoking in meeting halls and other public places, is it possible to reach a compromise between the rights of these two groups?

The efforts of some of the people who made the International Conference on Smoking and Reproductive Health the basis for this book will be evident as you read further. To my colleagues at Family Health International and elsewhere who helped inspire and shape this work, I extend my heartfelt appreciation. The extraordinary efforts of five persons deserve special mention: Russell Thomsen, for first suggesting the idea and his enthusiastic support during the initial planning; Philippa Charlton, for her editing and organizational skills and unflagging enthusiasm; Carol Williamson and Cathy Cunningham, for their skill, alacrity, and equanimity in typing and tracking manuscripts; and Ava Navin, for her editing craftsmanship.

Michael Rosenberg, MD, MPH
Chapel Hill, NC

I Smoking and Society

1 *Smoking and Reproductive Health*

Edward N. Brandt, Jr.

Clear scientific evidence indicates that smoking during pregnancy leads to reduced birth weight, with all of its sequelae, including lessened survival and physical and mental impairments of the infants who do survive. The smoke-exposed child is burdened with handicaps such as mental, cognitive, and physical defects that are never overcome. It is also clear that a woman who stops smoking, at least early in pregnancy, enhances the opportunity for her child to be healthy.

Cigarette smoking is clearly an addictive disorder. There are true physiologic withdrawal effects, and the craving for cigarettes has a physiologic basis. Like all addictive disorders, smoking is difficult to treat. The short-term success rate for pregnant women is low, and the recidivism rate is quite high. Indeed, there is evidence to indicate that women have a lower quit rate than men.

In the United States, and probably in most of the world, cigarette smoking is the number one preventable cause of death. It kills some 340,000 Americans each year by causing cancers of various sites, and it results in significant physical impairments, such as emphysema. Smoking women may shorten and impair their reproductive lives as well as undergo earlier menopause. Although many people have computed the economic cost of smoking in the United States, it is impossible to calculate the extent of human suffering.

The following data are from the United States; similar figures are available from throughout the world. A smoker is ten times more likely to die of lung cancer than a nonsmoker. Let us not forget, however, that lung cancer is only one of many cancers due to smoking cigarettes. Others are carcinomas of the larynx, oral cavity, and esophagus. In addition, smoking is strongly related to cancers of the bladder, pancreas, and kidneys. Indeed, in the United States, lung cancer has surpassed breast cancer as the leading cause of cancer death in women. Smoking during pregnancy, the topic of this book, leads to spontaneous abortion, prematurity, and low birth weight, as well as fetal and infant death. In addition, cigarette smoking in pregnancy is associated with sudden infant death syndrome and increased admission to neonatal intensive care units. Coronary artery disease is due in large part to cigarette smoking. Women who smoke and use oral contraceptives have ten times the risk of coronary artery disease of nonsmokers.

A number of controversies swirl around cigarette smoking. One has to do with the role of additives. Tobacco contains a number of organ-specific carcinogens, including nitrosamines and nitrosopiperidine, among others. The effects of those substances on the fetus are not known. Low-tar and low-nicotine cigarettes are developed by reducing the amount of tobacco and/or increasing the aeration of the tobacco while burning. Both these processes reduce the taste of cigarettes, so additives have been selected to give taste. The most common additive seems to be menthol, but the exact chemicals used are a competitive secret guarded zealously by manufacturers. Since relatively few toxicologic studies of substances burned at high temperatures have been done, it is not possible to determine whether additives increase the health risks of cigarette smoking.

A second controversy involves passive smoking, that is, the potential risk to nonsmokers from exposure to cigarette smoke. The most persistent recipient of passive smoking is the unborn child. Although the risk has not yet been defined except in the unborn child, clearly persons in a room with smokers inhale many of the same carcinogenic elements that smokers absorb. Children who live with one or more smoking parents have a far greater incidence of pulmonary and ear infections than do children who do not live in such an environment. In my judgment, passive smoking is a problem, and it does lead to a negative health impact on nonsmokers.

What can be done? In spite of the relatively low success rate of smoking cessation programs, therapeutic intervention is possible and does work. There are several important principles.

Cigarette smoking must be treated as an addiction similar to that with other drugs. Smoking cessation requires active intervention and the ability to tolerate the frustration of seeing patients quit and then start again and then quit and start again. It requires understanding and patience, and treatment must be individualized. No method of intervention works for all people. Not every patient is able to quit "cold turkey," and almost everyone requires a supportive environment. Communication experts have shown that scare tactics are not often effective in changing behavior. Telling a pregnant woman who smokes that she is harming and may kill her baby generally is not effective. Instead, she needs supportive encouragement from family members, friends, and co-workers as well as physicians and counselors. Cigarette smoking tends to be ritualistic; smokers tend to associate pleasurable aspects of smoking with specific times in their lives, such as after eating and during periods of anxiety and stress. Hence, withdrawal symptoms are most likely to occur during those periods. Positive reinforcement and encouragement are important during those times, when the positive aspects of stopping smoking can also be stressed. Specifically, as time passes, chronic nasal and laryngeal irritation will subside, taste will be enhanced, and exercise tolerance will improve. Since these changes tend to be gradual, the patient needs to be reminded of them frequently.

We can do many other things to promote a supportive and informative environment. For example, we can support local laws to restrict smoking in restaurants, workplaces, and other public places. Also, we can give greater visibility to the new warning labels on cigarette packs, of which one deals entirely with pregnancy and a second mentions it. Further, we can encourage all health associations and other groups to take positions against smoking and to ban smoking in meetings. It is especially important for our purposes here to encourage women's groups to take such stands. We can encourage the media to present more scientifically sound material on health generally and reproductive health in particular. Currently there is a great interest in health promotion, and one can hardly pick up a magazine or Sunday newspaper without seeing something about health. Although very little is published about health promotion in pregnancy or enough about smoking, cigarette ads are quite prominent.

We must not wait until a woman is pregnant to begin smoking cessation interventions. A woman who enters pregnancy having quit is much more likely to deliver a healthy baby than one who quits during pregnancy. Some therapeutic interventions can be used safely in nonpregnant women but may not be useful in pregnant women. For example, nicotine chewing gum or other forms of nicotine replacement in appropriate dosage can be safely used in nonpregnant women, but their safety in pregnancy has not been determined. Substances such as lobeline have also been found to be useful, but again, their safety in pregnancy has not been demonstrated.

My message can be summarized succinctly. First, cigarette smoking is a distinct health hazard that leads to marked physical impairments in the unborn, as well as death in both adults and fetuses. Second, it is a preventable and treatable condition. Third, women should stop smoking in pregnancy, or even better before pregnancy, within a total framework of good preventive medicine. Finally, we must all be aggressive in our pursuit of the goal of getting each woman, pregnant or not, to quit smoking. The Surgeon General of the US Public Health Service, Dr C. Everett Koop, has called for a smokefree society by the year 2000. Accepting that goal, however, is not enough. We must all work to make it happen. Each woman whom we convince to stop smoking represents a step in the right direction and can result in the saving of two lives—the mother and the baby.

2 *Smoking and Health: A 20-Year Reflection*

Donald R. Shopland

Last year was the anniversary of two major events in the history of cigarette smoking in the United States. The first event occurred 100 years earlier, when the first cigarette-making machine, invented by a young Virginian named James Bonsack, successfully ran for a full day in the factories of W. Duke and Company. This machine allowed large-scale production of factory cigarettes, which were uniform in quality and thus more appealing to the smoker. Although cigarette use was small compared with the use of other tobacco products before the turn of the century, this changed with the advent of the "blended" cigarette and with heavy promotion after the beginning of the twentieth century. In 1910, 9 billion cigarettes were smoked in the United States; in 1981 640 billion were smoked. In 1985 the estimate is for 595 billion—a reduction of about 7% compared with 1981, but still extremely high.

The second event occurred in January 1964, when the Advisory Committee to the Surgeon General issued its now-famous report on smoking and health. The committee's conclusion was that, "Cigarette smoking is a health hazard of sufficient importance in the United States to warrant appropriate remedial action." The committee based its opinion on evidence causally relating cigarette smoking to lung cancer, to cancer of the oral cavity, and to death from pulmonary emphysema. Smoking was also felt to be associated with other cancers and to be the most important cause of chronic bronchitis. The committee noted that women who smoked during pregnancy tended to have babies of lower birth weight but could not, based on the limited evidence then available, reach a causal conclusion.

If the first event ushered in the modern cigarette era, the second changed forever the way that we as a nation think about cigarette smoking as a socially accepted phenomenon. Until the release of the original Surgeon General's Advisory Committee report, smoking could only be characterized as a behavior that was being increasingly accepted by all segments of society. As a direct result of that first report, changes have occurred both in terms of overall smoking behavior and in that of young women, particularly those of childbearing age.

Among adults, cigarette smoking declined between 1955 and 1983 (Figure 2-1). Men had the most striking decrease, from over 50% in the mid-1950s to about 35% in 1983. A less dramatic change is seen in the percentage of smokers among women. In 1955, 25% of women smoked; this figure

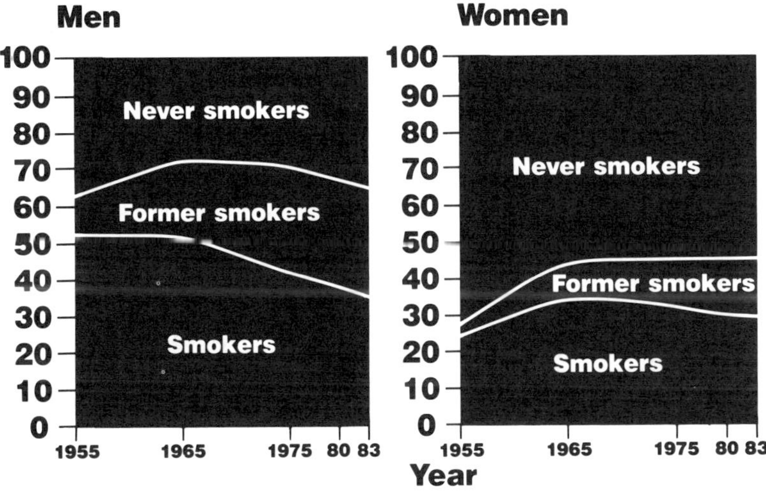

Figure 2-1 Percentage of smokers and nonsmokers, 1955-1983.

increased to 34% in the mid-1960s and decreased slightly to around 30% in 1983.

The pattern of former smokers among males and females also differs. The proportion of the adult male population who are ever-smokers (current or former smokers) has decreased from 75% in 1966 to 65% in 1983. Among women, however, the percentage of ever-smokers increased between 1955 and 1970, from 27.4% to 45.3%, and has since remained constant between 43% and 45%. Thus, the gap between the current smoking rates of men and women in the United States has narrowed considerably. This trend in smoking among adults is also evident in estimates of smoking among teenagers, as well as in surveys among high school students.

A greater proportion of teen-aged girls now smoke cigarettes than do teen-aged boys. Figures 2-2 and 2-3 depict changes in smoking behavior by birth cohorts of males and females.

The lifetime prevalence of cigarette smoking among men peaked in the cohort born from 1920 to 1929, with a rate of 77% ever-smokers (Figure 2-3); nearly 33% were still smoking at interview in 1983. Since these data were developed from cross-sectional estimates conducted when the men were 54 to 63 years of age, the lifetime prevalence of smoking probably exceeds this level because smokers are more likely not to have lived long enough to be interviewed. The smoking prevalence for all the male cohorts remains relatively high (nearly 70%) until the cohorts born after 1940, after which lifetime decreases.

In contrast to the situation among men, the lifetime prevalence of cigarette smoking among women did not peak until the cohorts born in 1930-1939 and 1940-1949 (Figure 2-4). The cohort of men born from 1920 to

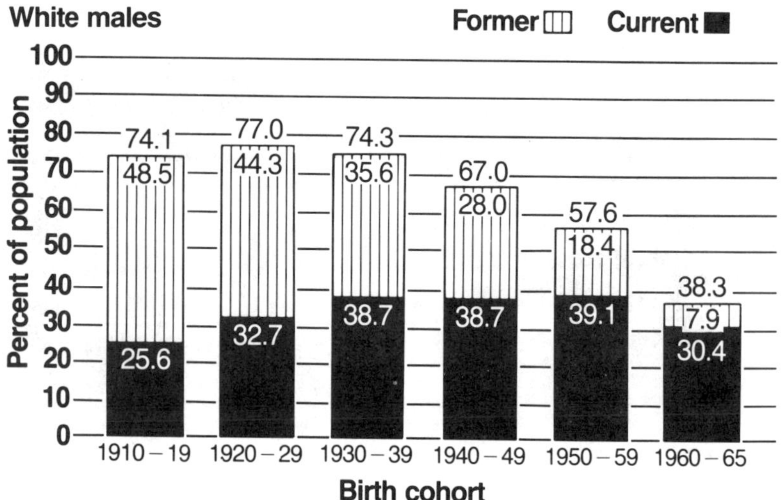

Figure 2-2 Lifetime prevalence of cigarette smoking by birth cohort (white males).

1929 had a peak prevalence rate of 77% ever-smokers; for women slightly over 47% ever-smokers are found in this cohort. The prevalence of lifetime history of smoking among males exceeds females in every birth cohort except for the youngest, those born after 1960.

Males and females also differ in the percentage who started regular

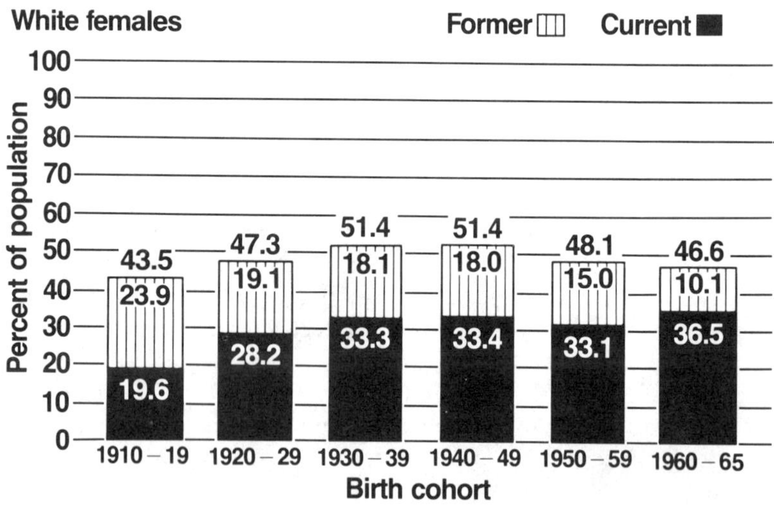

Figure 2-3 Lifetime prevalence of cigarette smoking by birth cohort (white females).

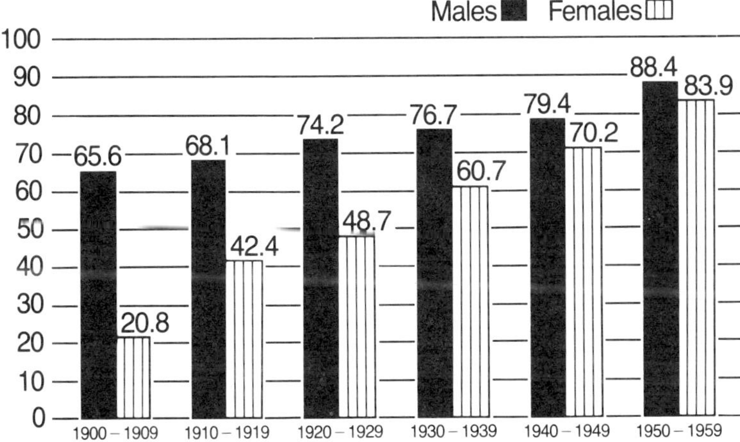

Figure 2-4 Percent smokers starting before age 20 years by birth cohort and sex.

cigarette smoking by age 20 (Figure 2-4). Progressively, however, the differences between initiation rates in males and females have narrowed, with little difference in the more contemporary cohorts in the percentage initiating smoking by age 20.

More recently (1983) the only major segment of our population showing an increase in smoking rates is young women. Women between the ages of 20 and 35, the childbearing years, have prevalence rates higher than those of previous cohorts of this age group. This finding is not unexpected, as this cohort was identified 10 to 12 years ago as having significantly greater use of cigarettes as teen-agers. These cohorts, some 10 years later, are now young adults. Unfortunately, these higher prevalence rates will be apparent again in another 20 to 25 years in the form of increased morbidity and mortality for various smoking-related diseases. Among women, lung cancer mortality is greater than that of breast cancer and is now the number one cancer killer for women. This trend may continue into the next century if future cohorts of young women do not change their behavior.

Public health officials must recognize, however, that quitting smoking is extremely difficult. A study by the National Center for Health Statistics in 1980 indicates that only about one of five pregnant women are able to stop smoking during their pregnancies. Unfortunately, many of these women resume smoking after pregnancy. Other studies are even less encouraging; for example, of persons who have suffered a heart attack and survived, only about half are able to quit permanently.

In a series of studies conducted by the Federal Trade Commission, smokers, while generally aware that their behavior is harmful, were not aware of the specific risks to their health caused by cigarette smoking. Federal legislation now requires that cigarette manufacturers print health warnings both on cigarette packs and in advertisements. Two labels specifically mention smoking during pregnancy: "Surgeon General's Warning: Smoking causes lung cancer, heart disease, and emphysema, and may complicate pregnancy"; and "Surgeon General's Warning: Smoking by pregnant women may result in fetal injury, premature birth, and low birth weight." These and other warnings replace the single warning that had been in use for almost 15 years.

Some good news is that preliminary data from a new study indicate that this year smoking rates may drop among both men and women. Data from the National Health Interview Survey show a sizeable reduction in the crude smoking rate of about 2% each for men and women. If these figures stand for the entire year, for the first time in over 40 years the smoking prevalence rates for the adult population may be at or below 30%.

3 *Tobacco Smoking Around the World*

Roberto Masironi

Since tobacco's discovery at the time when Columbus landed in the New World, it has played an increasing social and economic role in Western societies. In recent times, however, tobacco smoking has brought about a major health disaster to these societies. The spreading of the smoking habit, particularly cigarette smoking, has occurred like an epidemic; it first moved from one social group to another within very few Western countries then spread from country to country and from continent to continent, affecting developing countries as well. Worldwide, it has been calculated that about 600,000 new cases of lung cancer and over a million premature deaths each year occur because of cigarette smoking. Since the developing world constitutes a majority of the world's population, more and more of these deaths occur in developing countries.

Smoking-related diseases that are caused by widespread use of cigarettes are well known: they are myocardial and circulatory complications, cancer of the lung and other sites, chronic bronchitis and emphysema, and pregnancy complications. In developing countries, the use of other forms of tobacco brings about the same as well as other types of diseases, namely, cancer of the mouth associated with tobacco chewing, respiratory diseases associated with communal form of water pipe smoking, and increased susceptibility to bladder cancer in people affected by schistosomiasis.[1] Mention can be made here of the bidis, mostly smoked in Bangladesh, India and Nepal; chutta, which is common in parts of rural Nepal, as well as the water pipes, eg, hookah, goza, and narghila, which are smoked in Bangladesh, India, Nepal, Pakistan, Egypt, Tunisia and other countries of the Middle East. Tobacco chewing and snuff are widespread in many developing countries. The tobacco is chewed either alone or mixed with other vegetable and chemical products. In addition, the smoking materials used in some developing countries may be even more noxious than the materials smoked in the developed countries, as they yield much higher levels of toxic components, particularly tar and nicotine.

Trends in national consumption of tobacco generally precede and parallel national lung cancer rates. In some developing countries there has been an increase in cigarette consumption, but the per capita consumption is, fortunately, still much less than that for the developed countries. While overall tobacco consumption is slowing at 1.1% yearly in industrialized countries, it is rising by 2.1% a year in the Third World.

With increasing purchasing power the number of cigarettes smoked by such high numbers of people will inevitably increase, bringing in its wake increased morbidity and premature mortality. In some industrialized countries the impact of antismoking education on the amount smoked has been substantial. In countries such as Norway, Finland, the United Kingdom, and the United States, where smoking had been prevalent, the proportion of smokers has fallen and so, after a delay of a few years, has the average amount consumed. In some of these countries, too, the prevalence of smoking among women and young people, which had begun to increase many years after it had become common in men, has ceased to rise and begun to fall.

Where changes in smoking habits have occurred, they have begun first in the medical profession, extended to men and women in professional and other similar occupations, and are now spreading to other population strata. Unfortunately, an inverse pattern is evident in developing countries, where it is the professional men (and, more recently, women) who can afford to smoke cigarettes. Nevertheless, this steady progression through society holds out hope that smoking can be progressively diminished and largely eliminated, provided that smoking control and health education approaches are intensified.

The economics of tobacco production and the political pressure exerted by the tobacco industry are the major stumbling blocks in the way to eliminating this health-hazardous behavior. Developing countries, here again, find themselves at the losing end. A report made it clear that "...the developing countries are totally at the margin in the marketing decision process".[2] These countries gain only an insignificant share of the total profit made from tobacco growing as "their aggregate receipts from the tobacco industry are based, almost exclusively, on the demand response and the marketing decisions determined by the transnational tobacco companies, which are mostly foreign-based."[2] A more recent report on tobacco, issued by the Ministry of

Agriculture of Tanzania, also indicts the tobacco companies as being "in a position to dictate terms as they like, and often reject tobacco just for the sake of forcing the Tobacco Authority of Tanzania to reduce prices."[3] This report, and others as well, also point to the devastating environmental effects of tobacco growing. Approximately 1 hectare of forest is required to cure 1 hectare of tobacco. Disappearing woodlands are now an identifiable problem associated with tobacco growing in several developing countries, eg, Nepal, Sri Lanka, Pakistan, Tanzania, Sudan.

The lesson is obvious. The cigarette menace must be reduced as rapidly as possible and its spread to susceptible target groups—women and youth—must be prevented. The message is particularly relevant in a developing country situation. In the absence of strong and resolute action, we face the serious probability that the smoking epidemic will have affected the developing world within a few years, and a major avoidable public health problem will have been inflicted on countries least able to withstand it for the twin reasons of unscrupulous commercial enterprise and government inactivity. Failing immediate action, smoking diseases will appear in developing countries before infectious diseases and undernutrition have been controlled, and the gap between rich and poor countries will thus be further expanded.

REFERENCES

1. Ibrahim AS, Omar MS: *World Smoking Health* 1979;4:38-41.
2. United Nations Conference on Trade and Development: *Marketing and Distribution of Tobacco.* United Nations, Geneva, 1978.
3. Price Policy Recommendations for the July 1983 Agricultural Price Review: Annex A, Tobacco R1/83, by Marketing Development Bureau Ministry of Agriculture, United Republic of Tanzania, Dar Es Salaam, 1983, p 15.

4 *Cell to Organism: Tobacco's Influence on Development*

R.T. Ravenholt

When optimal gametes combine to form an optimal zygote and the resultant organism develops in an optimal intrauterine environment, the result is a healthy newborn infant. There are, however, many deleterious agents in the general and uterine environments which assail germ cells and the developing organism and which may deviate germ and somatic cells from their primeval purposes.

Tobacco smoke entering the lungs of pregnant women contains polonium 210—an alpha particle-emitting form of ionizing radiation—plus hundreds of chemical mutagens[1-3] which also enter the maternal and fetal circulation.[4,5] The question of interest is thus not *whether* smoking alters the normal development of cells, but rather *the extent* of these changes and whether they are corrected by the developing cell or canceled by fetal death.

METHOD OF STUDY

As part of a review of relevant literature, data were reexamined from an earlier study in Seattle on the effects of smoking upon reproduction as measured by changes in fetal deaths, livebirth weights, and sex ratios.[6,7] In addition, data were reviewed from closely associated studies of parental smoking in relation to congenital malformations, mental retardation, and childhood leukemia among offspring.[8,9] A detailed description of the methods of these studies has been published.[7]

These earlier data were collected with meticulous concern for quantitative measurement of the preconceptional smoking experience of mothers and fathers and of the mothers' smoking experience during pregnancy, facili,tated by a charting technique (Figure 4-1).[7] Such careful measurement of lifetime and gestational smoking experience in relation to pregnancy outcome is essential for defining the effects of smoking on reproduction. Much of the uncertainty and confusion that still exists concerning effects of maternal smoking derives from inadequate quantitative measure,ment of smoking experience in many studies.

RESULTS

Data from the Seattle study of 2023 liveborn infants (Figure 4-2) show the impact of maternal smoking on the birth weight and male-to-female ratio of offspring. Clearly, the extent of maternal smoking during pregnancy is a much more powerful determinant of birth weight and male-to-female ratio of offspring than is the extent of maternal smoking before conception. The average birth weight of infants born to mothers who smoked heavily during pregnancy was reduced by approximately 0.5 lb, and the male-to-female ratio was several percent less (49.4% males) for infants born to heavily smoking mothers (4000+ cigarettes during pregnancy) than for infants born to nonsmoking mothers (53% males). This finding, suggesting greater losses of male fetuses in women smoking heavily during pregnancy, is buttressed by similar findings by Asmussen.[10] To measure the effects of parental smoking on the male-to-female ratio of liveborn offspring, the extent of maternal smoking during pregnancy must be measured separately from maternal and paternal smoking before conception.

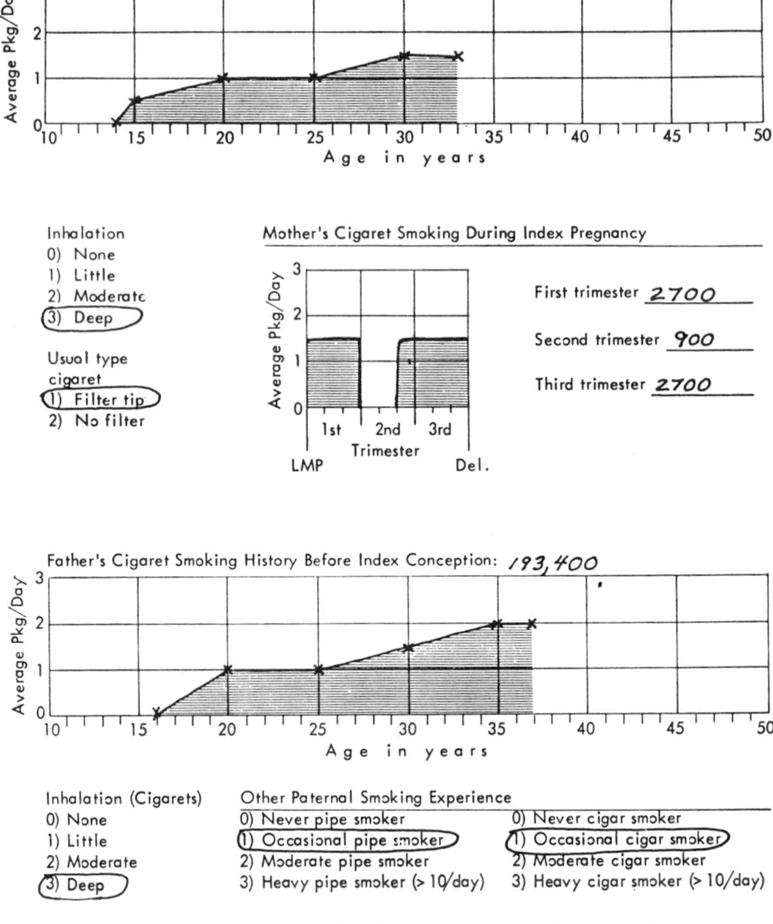

Figure 4-1 Parental preconceptional smoking experience. Lifetime consumption of cigarettes is calculated by counting the number of rectangles or fractions thereof under the charted line(s) and multiplying by 36,500. (Reproduced with permission from Ravenholt et al.[7])

In 1981, with the help of the Community Health Department of Clark County, Nevada, an analogous survey was done of mothers delivering liveborn infants in Las Vegas-Clark County, Nevada.[11] The average smoking mother smoked 50,800 cigarettes before the index pregnancy. Twenty-eight percent of mothers smoked during pregnancy, and the average maternal smoker, smoking 4100 cigarettes, had a baby weighing 6.9 lb, compared with the 7.8 lb average weight of infants born to nonsmoking mothers. Thus, the average birth weight deficit of smoke-exposed infants was 0.9 lb—consid-

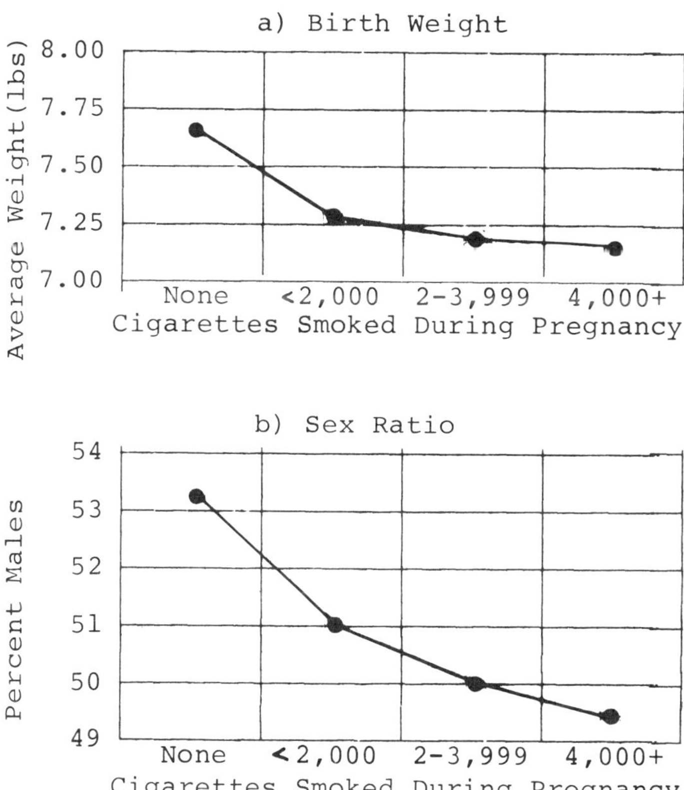

Figure 4-2 Effects of maternal smoking upon birth weight and sex ratio of liveborn offspring, Seattle, 1964. (Reproduced with permission from Ravenholt et al.[7])

erably more than the average birth weight deficit found for liveborn infants of smokers in Seattle 17 years earlier.

The growth impairment effect of maternal smoking remains consistently strong after the data are adjusted for sex of infant, duration of gestation, size and age of parents, and birth order of offspring. That maternal smoking can also sometimes kill the fetus is a well-demonstrated fact from many studies.[12,13] Spontaneous abortion rates usually increase by at least a third in pregnant smokers and double for women smoking heavily during pregnancy.[13,14] Of even greater importance than the killing effects of smoking on fetuses lost by abortion and perinatal death are its maiming effects on surviving infants. Findings from the Seattle studies demonstrate increases in childhood leukemia (Table 4-1) among offspring of mothers smoking most heavily during pregnancy. Additional studies are needed for better measure-

Table 4-1
Condition of Offspring by Smoking Experience of Mothers During Pregnancy

No. Cigarettes Smoked by Mother During Pregnancy	No. Births	Normal	Condition of Offspring Down's Syndrome	Other Mental	Childhood Leukemia
None	1377	90.6%	1.9%	5.2%	2.3%
< 2000	271	88.9%	1.8%	7.4%	1.8%
2000-3999	215	91.2%	0.9%	6.0%	1.9%
4000 +	381	88.7%	1.3%	5.8%	4.2%

Data from Ravenholt et al.[7,8]

ment of the kinds and numbers of childhood cancers attributable to maternal smoking.

DISCUSSION

Sufficient evidence has accumulated to indicate that maternal smoking is a hazard to the health and life of mother and child. Approximate annual consequences of 1 million pregnant women smoking in the United States (1980) include: 100,000+ fetal deaths, 4000 infant deaths, 5000 congenital malformations, and 200,000+ infants who are perceptibly growth-impaired.[15]

Failure of the obstetrician to accurately ascertain lifetime and gestational maternal smoking practices and take appropriate action to protect the vulnerable fetus therefrom may be viewed as just as serious a breach of acceptable practice as failure to identify gestational anemia, hypertension, or an Rh problem. In addition to having each patient chart her lifetime and current smoking experience[16] at her initial antenatal visit, a test for thiocyanate in blood, urine, or saliva should be made at least once.[17]

A misdirection of medical and social action has occurred in recent decades, with neonatologists applying ever more sophisticated and expensive measures in attempting to save the least viable products of gestational disasters rather than intervening early to ensure each fetus a smoke-free uterine environment.

CONCLUSIONS

The combination of an alpha particle-emitting radioisotope (polonium 210) with an addictive substance (nicotine) has made tobacco the foremost human poison of the twentieth century.

This poison is currently being administered with impunity by cigarette companies and addicted pregnant women to approximately 1 million embryonic Americans annually, with tragic consequences. In addition to causing approximately 100,000 fetal deaths and 4000 infant deaths each year in the United States,[18] maternal smoking causes congenital malformations of an estimated 5000 surviving infants and perceptible growth impairment of several hundred thousand infants. For those young who somehow survive the intrauterine tobacco gauntlet seemingly unscathed, there still lurks the specter of leukemia and other malignancies of childhood and increased adult cancers and cardiovascular diseases throughout a shortened lifetime of diminished health and vigor.

REFERENCES

1. Radford EP, Hunt VR: Polonium 210: A volatile radioelement in cigarettes. *Science* 1964;143:247-249.
2. Ravenholt RT: Circulating mutagens from smoking. *N Engl J Med* 1982;307:312.
3. Ames BN: Identifying environmental chemicals causing mutations and cancer. *Science* 1979;204:587-593.
4. Everson RB: Individuals transplacentally exposed to maternal smoking may be at increased cancer risk in adult life. *Lancet* 1980;2:123-127.
5. Asmussen I: Ultrastructure of the villi and fetal capillaries in placentas from smoking and nonsmoking mothers. *Br J Obstet Gynaecol* 1980;87:239-245.
6. Ravenholt RT, Levinski MJ: Smoking during pregnancy. *Lancet* 1965;1:961.
7. Ravenholt RT, Levinski MJ, Nellist D, et al: Effects of smoking upon reproduction. *Am J Obstet Gynecol* 1966;96:267-281.
8. Ravenholt RT, Clark O, Levinski MJ, et al: The role of tobacco in cellular deviation. Presented to the American Public Health Association, Chicago, October 1965.
9. Ravenholt RT: Smoking and reproduction, in Proceedings of the First International Congress of Maternal and Neonatal Health. Manila, November 6, 1981.
10. Asmussen I: Effects of maternal smoking on the fetal cardiovascular system. *Cardiovasc Med* 1979;4:777-790.
11. Ravenholt RT, Ravenholt OH, Payne D, et al: Multi-state birth surveys. Presented to the Annual Meeting of the American Public Health Association. Los Angeles, November 4, 1981. Published in part in *Morbidity and Mortality Weekly Report* 1982;31:61-63.
12. Coleman S, Piotrow PT, Rinehart W: *Tobacco—Hazards to Health and Human Reproduction.* Population Reports Series L, No. 1. Baltimore, Johns Hopkins University, 1979.
13. US Dept of Health and Human Services: The Health Consequences of Smoking for Women: A Report of the Surgeon General. Government Printing Office, 1980.
14. Kline J, Stein ZA, Susser M, et al: Smoking: a risk factor for spontaneous abortion. *N Engl J Med* 1977;297:793-796.
15. Ravenholt RT: Addiction Mortality in the United States, 1980: Tobacco, alcohol and other substances. *Popul Dev Rev* 1984;10:697-724.

16. Ravenholt RT: Charting lifetime smoking experience. *World Health Forum* 1982;3:104.
17. Meberg A, Sande H, Foss OP, et al: Smoking during pregnancy—effects on the fetus and on thiocyanate levels in mother and baby. *Acta Pediatr Scand* 1979;68:547-552.
18. Ravenholt RT: Tobacco's impact on twentieth century US mortality patterns. *Am J Prevent Med* 1985;1:4-17.

5 *Advertising and Marketing of Cigarettes to Women*

Virginia L. Ernster

Despite basic product similarity and a deadly common denominator, different cigarette brands are advertised so as to appeal to a broad spectrum of distinct and desirable personality types. The positive imagery used by the tobacco industry suggests that women who smoke are sexually attractive, exciting, liberated, ambitious, athletic, self-indulgent, and fun-loving.

Featuring women in cigarette promotions goes back to the 1880s, when almost all smokers were men. Together with the purchase of Duke cigarettes came coupons featuring voluptuous women athletes, including a tennis player, a horsewoman, a swimmer, and a bullfighter.[1] Targeting women directly as smokers began in the 1920s, when it was still considered inappropriate to picture a woman holding a cigarette, as in a romantic Chesterfield advertisement in which a woman is quoted as saying "Blow some my way" to her smoking male companion. A successful advertising campaign, begun in the latter half of the 1920s, sounded a theme that has since become a hallmark of cigarette advertising directed at women: the association of smoking with slenderness. It read: "The fearless shadow that threatens the modern figure.... When tempted, reach for a Lucky instead" (Figure 5-1).

The association of sexual desirability with cigarette smoking was well established by the 1930s. Advertisements of the period also featured the testimonials of prominent socialites. The first ad to appear in the *Ladies Home Journal*, in 1933, is captioned "Tea at the Ritz." The script reads: "Women are flavor experts--naturally they choose the best..." and concludes, "That's why they pick Camels."[2]

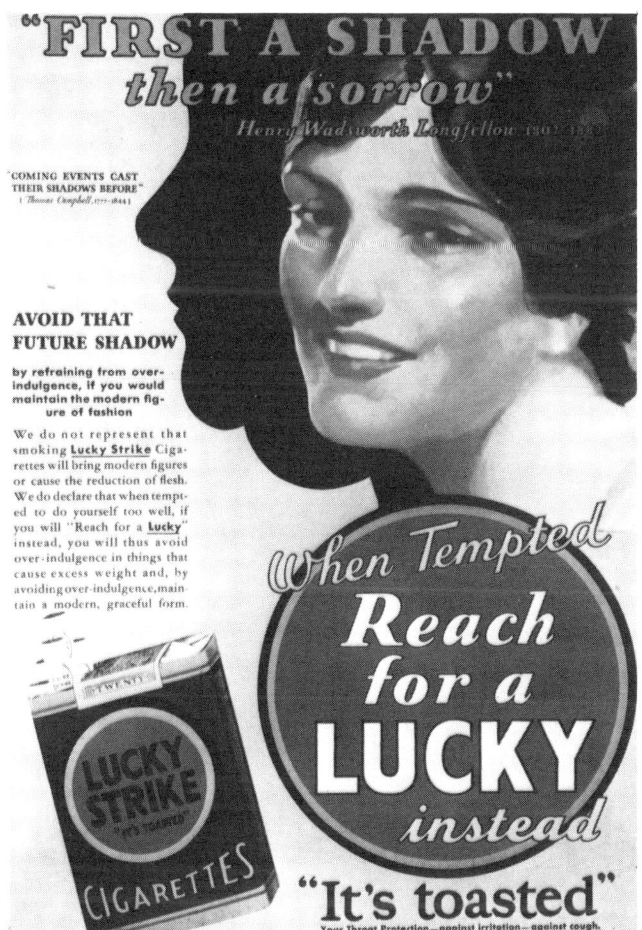

Figure 5-1

During World War II, cigarette advertising directed at women featured patriotic themes and celebrities, including Betty Grable and Rosalind Russell, the latter dressed as an air warden.[3] A 1943 ad featured a female riveter, with a cigarette hanging out of her mouth and a pack in her overalls pocket (Figure 5-2). An inset stated, "Women at work. It is estimated that 15,000,000 women are employed in U.S. industry today," and the text below added, "When you're doing a bang-up job, you want a bang-up smoke."[4] The hard-working independent images of women ended with the war, as women in the ads became wives and lovers. A telegram set in the upper corner of one ad read, "Just landed, be home today. Love Dick," and a woman wearing a dressing gown ponders, "He's coming home...Everything's going to be just the way he'll want it. His easy chair...his slippers...and his Chesterfields."[5]

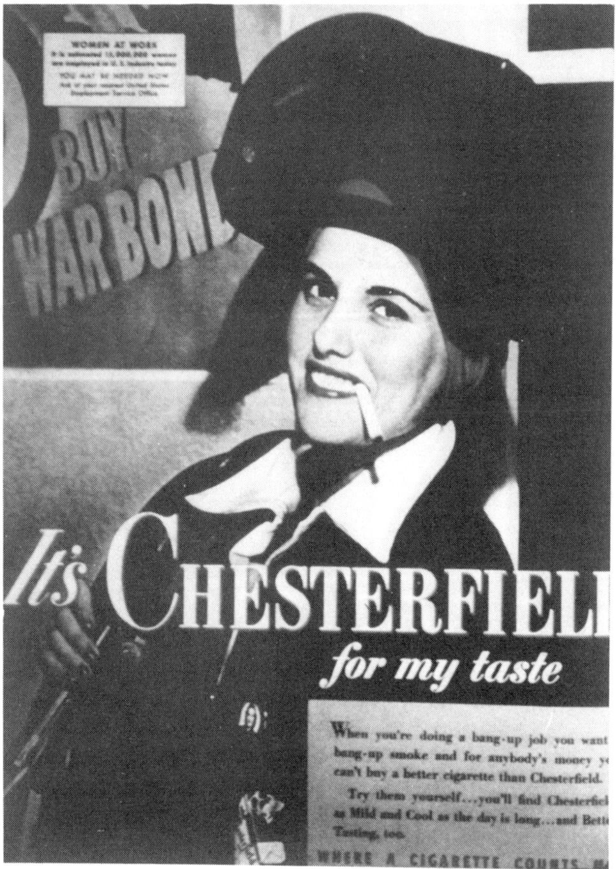

Figure 5-2

In 1964, the US tobacco industry adopted its own cigarette advertising code. The code, intended to apply to broadcast advertising, stated that cigarette manufacturers intended to avoid advertising directed to young persons and to avoid advertising representing cigarette smoking as "essential to social prominence, distinction, success, or sexual attraction"; and to refrain from depicting smokers engaged in sports or other activities "requiring stamina or athletic conditioning beyond that of normal recreation."[6,7] Although the code officially ended in 1970, it is still cited as a standard of industry behavior.[8] Two decades later many, if not most, cigarette advertisements violate the spirit of the code, with scenes depicting vigorous sporting activities, images that epitomize social success, and sexually alluring models.

A major arena for cigarette advertising is women's magazines (see Table 5-1). There is strong evidence that the content of these publications is re-

Table 5-1
Cigarette Advertising in Major America Women's Magazines, January–May 1985, and Comparison with January–May 1984

Magazine	A Average No. of Cigarette Ad Pages per Issue	1985 B Cigarette Advertising Revenues	C Cigarette Advertising as Percent of Total Ad Revenues	1984 D Cigarette Advertising as Percent of Total Ad Revenues	Change From 1984 to 1985 in Cigarette Advertising as Percent of Total Ad Revenues
Better Homes & Gardens	10.4	$4,705,567	9.28	12.0	−23.3
Cosmopolitan	11.0	2,704,580	6.9	7.4	−6.8
Essence	7.0	620,346	8.9	10.3	−13.6
Family Circle	8.1	4,529,680	7.8	14.1	−44.6
Glamour	10.6	2,177,543	7.2	7.3	−1.4
Good Housekeeping	0.0	0	0.0	0.0	–
Harper's Bazaar	7.3	895,185	7.0	8.5	−17.6
Ladies Home Journal	10.8	3,216,873	10.6	13.2	−20.0
Mademoiselle	7.7	1,043,243	7.4	5.8	+27.6
McCall's	9.8	3,627,264	11.4	14.4	−20.8
Ms	3.0	173,624	6.7	7.8	−14.1
New Woman	8.4	588,000	16.5	17.4	−5.2
Redbook	11.1	2,918,413	13.6	16.2	-16.0
Vogue	9.3	1,340,971	4.7	5.0	-6.0
Woman's Day	9.4	4,519,285	10.3	12.0	−14.2
Working Mother	9.0	668,430	13.3	8.3	+60.2
Working Women	7.2	655,300	8.0	10.4	−23.1

Data from *Leading National Advertisers. Magazine and Class Totals,* May 1985, Publishers Information Bureau, 1985.
Based on data in columns C and D.

strained in reporting smoking-related issues because of the heavy dependence on cigarette advertising revenues.[7,10] The paucity of reporting on smoking and women's health has been documented in American women's magazines by Whelan et al[11] and Dale.[12] In a well-,publicized report produced by the British Medical Association, Jacobson and Amos[13] recently observed that, while there appears to be improvement in coverage of smoking and health in British women's magazines during the last few years, only 37% of women's magazines had recently covered or planned to cover the subject. The authors concluded, "those who derived above average revenue from cigarettes were much less likely to devote any major attention to smoking and health."[13]

Magazines are not passive recipients of cigarette advertising revenues. The *U.S. Tobacco and Candy Journal* regularly carries ads from such publications as *People* and *Time* magazines soliciting cigarette accounts, with such slogans as "Light Up Your Sales With The People Generation"[14] or "Where there's smoke...there's a hot market for cigarette advertisers in *Time*."[15] The text of the ad from which the latter slogan was drawn states that women are showing substantial growth in cigarette volume and invites calls to *Time*'s "Tobacco Category Manager," whose name and telephone number are provided.

Close to $2 billion are spent annually by the tobacco industry to advertise and promote cigarettes in the United States.[16] Much of this money is devoted to linking cigarettes with socially valued activities. The major jazz festival in the country is sponsored by and carries the name of Kool cigarettes. Programs for stage plays and musicals throughout the country are underwritten by cigarette advertising. The largest grant in corporate exhibition-giving history ($3 million) was from Philip Morris, Inc to the Metropolitan Museum of Art to underwrite the acclaimed Vatican Art Exhibit in the United States during the early 1980s.[17] Philip Morris also helps to sponsor the Joffrey Ballet, and in its corporate ads uses the slogan "It takes art to make a company great."[18] Becoming patrons of the arts enhances corporate image, while perhaps silencing critics in high places.

Cigarette promotions have also been placed in the world of fashion. The reader of popular publications turns the pages from a frank cigarette ad to a fashion spread, and the images blend to create an impression linking cigarettes and style. That union was consummated with the introduction of the Ritz brand of cigarettes by R.J. Reynolds Industries, Inc. Test-marketed in several areas of the United States in 1985, each pack and individual Ritz cigarette bears the logo of designer Yves St. Laurent[19] (Figure 5-3). In the world of sports, professional women's tennis tournaments in the United States carry the name of their sponsor, Virginia Slims cigarettes. Free cigarette samples are distributed at the entrance to the tennis matches.

In another attempt to associate itself with valued institutions, the Tobacco Institute recently collaborated with the National Association of State Boards of Education to produce a booklet entitled *Helping Youth Decide*. The

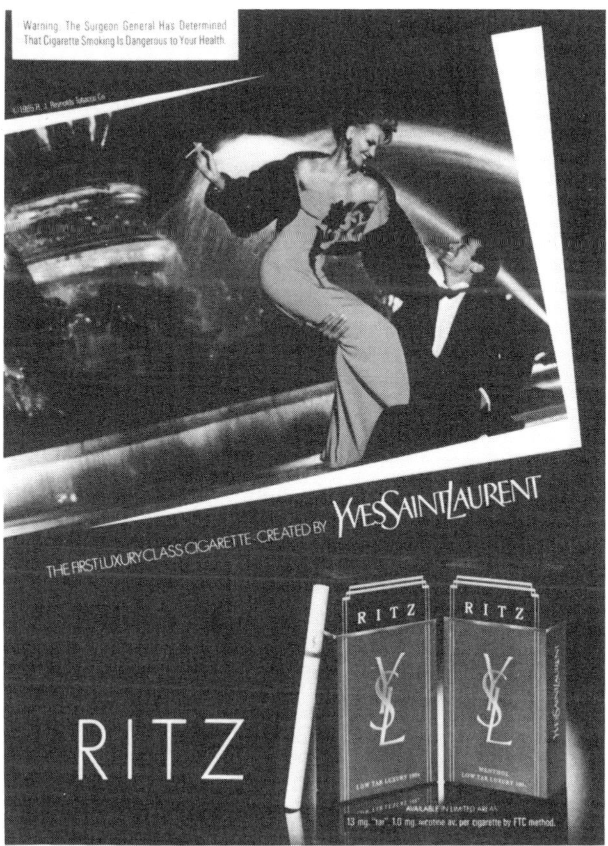

Figure 5-3

inside jacket of the booklet reads, "This publication of the National Association of State Boards of Education was made possible by the Tobacco Institute. The Tobacco Institute is an association of cigarette manufacturers who—as a matter of long-time policy and practice—believe that smoking is an adult custom. Simply put, the people who make cigarettes do not want young people smoking them." The booklet has been publicized in ads in national magazines and newspapers. The ad in the June 1985 issue of *Better Homes & Gardens*, captioned "How to Get Your Teenager Talking to You," appeared on the page immediately before a feature piece entitled "Parenting: New Approaches to Old Discipline Problems."

The youthful-looking models in many of the ads suggest that cigarette companies are keenly aware that the habit of regular cigarette smoking is usually established by the age of 15 or 16 years and that recruitment of future smokers must begin early. Youth-oriented promotional efforts include cigarette distribution near rock concerts,[20] the sponsoring by Camel cigarettes of activities for vacationing college students,[21] and the multiple appearances of Marlboro in the movie Superman II.[22] To reassure the public, the Tobacco Institute and R.J. Reynolds have produced a stream of public relations ads. One of these poses the question, "Do cigarette companies want kids to smoke?" The text answers, "No. As a matter of policy. No. As a matter of practice. No. As a matter of fact. No."[23]

Given the mixed messages and the relative lack of media attention to smoking issues, it is perhaps not surprising that a 1980 Roper Poll found that 47% of women were unaware that smoking during pregnancy increases the risk of "losing the baby before or during birth."[8] Public awareness may change as a result of new warning labels that began to appear on cigarette packages and ads in October 1985. One reads, "Surgeon General's Warning: Smoking causes lung cancer, heart disease, emphysema, and may complicate pregnancy." Another focuses specifically on pregnancy: "Surgeon General's Warning: Smoking by pregnant women may result in fetal injury, premature birth, and low birth weight." These warnings occupy a small corner of space on ads in which healthy, appealing, self-confident women loom large. A discordant mix of negative and positive messages continues to characterize the sociocultural milieu of smoking for women. The widespread cigarette advertising and promotion may help to explain the relatively high prevalence of smoking by women in the face of the myriad health risks summarized in other parts of this book.

REFERENCES

1. *Life*, July 26, 1954, pp 2-3.
2. *Ladies Home Journal*, May 1933, p 56.
3. *Better Homes & Gardens*, October 1942, back cover.
4. *Better Homes & Gardens*, March 1943, back cover.
5. *Better Homes & Gardens*, October 1944, back cover.
6. Friedman KM: *Public Policy and the Smoking-Health Controversy: A Comparative Study*. Lexington, Mass, Lexington Books, 1975, p 44.
7. Cummins K: The cigarette makers: How they get away with murder. *The Washington Monthly*, April 1984, pp 14-24; March 1985, pp 48-54.
8. Myers ML, Iscoe C, Jennings C, et al: *Staff Report on the Cigarette Advertising Investigation*. Washington, Federal Trade Commission, May 1981, Chapter 5, pp 12-13.
9. *Leading National Advertisers. Magazines and Class Totals*. May 1985, New York Publishers Information Bureau, 1985.
10. Warner K: Cigarette advertising and media coverage of smoking and health. *N Engl J Med* 1985;312:384-388.
11. Whelan EM, Sheridan MJ, Meister KA, et al: Analysis of coverage of tobacco hazards in women's magazines. *J Public Health Policy* 1981;2:28-35.

12. Dale KC: ACSH Survey: Which magazines report the hazards of smoking? *ACSH News & Views* May/June 1982; pp 8-10.
13. Jacobson B, Amos A: When smoke gets in your eyes: Cigarette advertising policy and coverage of smoking and health in women's magazines. British Medical Association Professional Division, London, May 1985, p 24.
14. *U.S. Tobacco and Candy Journal*, May 9-29, 1985, p 5.
15. *U.S. Tobacco and Candy Journal*, August 1-21, 1985, p 20. 16. Federal Trade Commission: *Report to Congress Pursuant to the Federal Cigarette Labeling and Advertising Act for the Years 1982-1983*. Washington, Federal Trade Commission, June 1985.
17. Treasures from the see. *San Francisco Focus*, September 1983, p 10.
18. *U.S. Tobacco and Candy Journal*, March 28 - April 17, 1985, pp 8-9.
19. Gloede WF: RJR puts on the Ritz. *Advertising Age*, January 21, 1985, pp 1,78.
20. ABC News 20/20: Growing up in smoke. Transcript of program broadcast on October 20, 1983.
21. Where the bucks are. *Time*, April 4, 1983, pp 58,60.
22. Magnus P: Superman and the Marlboro woman: The lungs of Lois Lane. *NY State J Med* 1985;85:342-343.
23. *Time*, September 19, 1983, pp 10-11.

6 *Smoking and the Women's Movement*

Carol J. R. Hogue, Stuart M. Berman

The women's movement and smoking among women are inextricably intertwined. Both promoters and opponents of cigarettes recognize that smoking is a feminist issue.[1] This paper examines the reasons for the relationship between smoking and feminism and the roles spokeswomen for the women's movement are assuming for communicating antismoking messages to other women.

Although advertisers were perhaps the first to realize the impact of feminism on women's smoking habits, smoking is also identified as a feminist issue by health promoters, in part because women are rapidly catching up to men in smoking-related deaths, especially deaths from lung cancer.[1] The rise in lung cancer mortality in women is closely associated with the ever-decreasing age of smoking initiation among women.[2] More teen-aged girls than boys are smokers.[3] In addition, smoking jeopardizes the health of mothers and lays the burden of caring for less healthy infants most heavily on women already burdened by lives of social deprivation—the poorly educated,[4-6] the unmarried,[5,6] and teen-agers.[5,6]

With respect to the reproductive health problems of smoking women, Jacobson, in her 1982 book *The Ladykillers*,[7] comments, "[a] peculiar silence—almost a resistance—surrounds the question of smoking among women's organizations. As far as the women's movement is concerned, smoking is someone else's problem." Her documentation of the silence at that time included a lack of attention to smoking in the early editions of the key health handbook, *Our Bodies, Ourselves*; no reference to the problem of smoking by women in the 40-page submission to the 1979 Kennedy hearings on women's health made by the National Organization for Women (NOW); the fact that the only organization to raise the issue of rising lung cancer rates among women was the American Cancer Society; and lack of "a formal position on smoking" or antismoking programs by the National Women's Health Network and local women's health organizations. (At NOW's last annual meeting a resolution to ban cigarette smoking and cigarette advertising at their meetings was introduced. It was defeated after an amendment to ban alcohol as well was added.) Jacobson concludes this section;

> [the] Birmingham Women's Health Group seemed to sum up the prevailing attitude among many British women's groups: 'When we read your letter there was a great reluctance in the group to spend a whole meeting discussing smoking. Most members (despite being smokers themselves) felt there were more important issues to discuss.[7]

In 1985, Arthur Holleb's editorial in *CA*[1] called on *NOW*, the National Women's Health Network, other women's health collectives, women's magazines, and consumer groups "to speak out against the manipulation of young women by cigarette manufacturers and against cigarette smoking in general." Responses to this editorial by several leaders in the women's movement[8] suggest that the movement is now divided between two positions: that held by the women's political movement and that held by the women's health movement. The political arm is uninvolved, while the health arm is involved in public education, activism, and individual counseling. Activities undertaken by members of the women's health movement include organizing antismoking topics at the Fourth Regional Conference on Women and Medicine (April 1986), picketing by the Women's Health Network of a Virginia Slims-sponsored tennis tournament at George Washington University on January 12, 1985, and the incorporation of several antismoking messages in the new edition of *Our Bodies,Ourselves*.[9]

Concern for all women who smoke is reflected in the philosophy expressed in the new edition of *Our Bodies*, *Ourselves*,[9] the health handbook published by the Boston Women's Health Book Collective. "It is a major aim of the feminist movement to make the crucial tools for health and survival available to everyone."[9] This concern is balanced by strong encouragement to stop smoking. "It is hard to stop smoking. But it is also possible—and it is one of the biggest favors we will ever do for ourselves and our health."[9] In addition, self-help aids are listed along with organizations, books, and audiovisual aids, including the movie, *The Feminine Mistake*. This film is described as "a straightforward presentation of the dangers of cigarette smoking aimed primarily at young women."

Compared with *WomanCare*, published by the American Medical Association in 1984,[10] *Our Bodies, Ourselves* presents more facts about smoking. Moreover, *Our Bodies, Ourselves* presents a greater amount of information on how to stop smoking in a more encouraging manner. The *Ms. Guide to a Woman's Health*[11] contains more antismoking material than does *WomanCare*, but the treatment is somewhat more superficial than the presentation in *Our Bodies, Ourselves*.

Smoking is a feminist issue because cigarette advertisers misuse the liberation message, because the reproductive health risks borne by women smokers are not shared by male smokers, and because the burden of smoking-related maternal and infant morbidity falls most heavily on women who are already disadvantaged. The women's health movement actively opposes smoking among women, but feminists have yet to make the connection between disadvantaged mothers and their risk of raising less healthy infants as a result of their greater tendency to smoke. Moreover, the women's political movement has yet to abjure cigarette advertisements. Spokeswomen for the women's movement are active proponents of reproductive health and are thus a potentially potent force for communicating to women the adverse effects of smoking on reproductive health.

REFERENCES

1. Holleb AI: Lung cancer: A feminist issue, editorial. *CA-Cancer J Clinicians* 1985;35:125-126.
2. US Dept of Health and Human Services: *The Health Consequences of Smoking for Women. A report of the Surgeon General.* Government Printing Office, 1980, pp 28-33.
3. Feldman RD, Feldman RP: The prevalence of cigarette smoking among teenagers: An 18-year study. *J Indiana State Med Assoc* 1983;76:456-459.
4. Kleinman JC, Madans JH: The effects of maternal smoking, physical stature, and educational attainment on the incidence of low birthweight. *Am J Epidemiol* 1985;121:843-855.
5. Dalaker K, Grunfeld B, Jansen A: Smoking in pregnancy. *J Oslo City Hosp* 1984;34:21-27.
6. Schramm W: Smoking and pregnancy outcome. *Mo Med* 1980;77:619-626.
7. Jacobson B: *The Ladykillers: Why Smoking Is a Feminist Issue.* New York, Continuum Publishing Co, 1982, pp 78-79.

8. McCormack P: Groups fume over warning women of smoking dangers. Chicago, *Daily Southtown Economist*, March 7, 1985.
9. Boston Women's Health Book Collective: *The New Our Bodies, Ourselves*. New York, Simon & Schuster, 1985.
10. American Medical Association: *The American Medical Association's Straight-Talk No-Nonsense Guide to WomanCare*. New York, Random House, 1984.
11. Cooke CW, Dworkin S: *The Ms. Guide to a Woman's Health*. New York, Berkley Books, 1979.

II Contraception, Conception, and Development

7 *Smoking, Oral Contraceptives, and Other Risk Factors for Atherosclerotic Heart Disease*

Jeffrey A. Perlman, Ronald M. Krauss, Rose Ray, Ronnette Russell-Briefel, Trena Ezzati, Greg Lieberknecht

Despite the well-established association between smoking, *current* use of oral contraceptives (OCs), and vascular disease, little is known about how smoking and the pill alter the long--term risk of atherosclerotic heart disease in older, past pill users. Concern has been raised about joint exposure to the progestational component of the pill and smoking, since both exposures adversely affect lipid metabolism.[1-3] These effects include elevation of serum total cholesterol and LDL cholesterol and reduction of HDL cholesterol, all of which independently predict atherosclerotic disease.[4-6]

This chapter examines how smoking and OC use alter a young woman's risk profile for heart disease. Data from a large prospective study are used to evaluate the interaction of progestin dose, smoking, and other risk factors. Subsequently, data from the second National Health and Nutrition Examination Survey (NHANES II) are presented to compare the national prevalence of moderate- and high-risk heart disease profiles among the nation's population of OC users and nonusers and to examine how smoking influences these findings.

MATERIALS AND METHODS

The Walnut Creek Contraceptive Drug Study (WCCDS) is a 10-year prospective study, conducted between 1968 and 1972, of 16,638 women aged 18 through 54 years. At the first study visit, medical and contraceptive histories were taken, physical examinations performed, and biochemical tests taken. This evaluation was repeated when a woman returned to Kaiser for her annual checkup or medical attention. Detailed study methodology is documented elsewhere.[7-9] Additional determinations of cholesterol and triglycerides were performed on 5005 women in 1975 and 1976. From these specimens, cholesterol and triglycerides were measured enzymatically in plasma precipitated with manganese chloride and heparin solution. High density cholesterol and triglyceride were measured in the supernate using a

Technicon AAII procedure. VLDL cholesterol was measured as 20% of the referrent triglyceride concentration. Specimens were excluded from this analysis for women who were taller than 70in or shorter than 57in, weighed more than 40% over Metropolitan Life tables' ideal, had a history of diabetes or having more than two alcoholic drinks each day, were over age 40 years, or used non-contraceptive estrogens. This analysis is thus composed of 209 current OC users, 1123 past OC users, and 192 never users.

Linear regression was used to assess the impact of smoking and hormone dose on lipoprotein measures while controlling for other risk factors for heart disease. The various cholesterol values (mg/dL) were the dependent variable for each model while age, body mass index (lb/in^2), systolic and diastolic blood pressure, family history of heart disease (yes/no), smoking status (yes/no), and dose of estrogen and norethindrone served as independent variables. Thus, in the HDL model, a statistically significant slope of -2 for norethindrone indicates that for each mg of norethindrone, HDL is lowered by 2 mg/dL, given that all other risk factors are held constant.

NHANES II is a national morbidity survey of the civilian, noninstitutionalized population of the United States. The survey involves full medical history and physical examinations, medicine and medical-care use questionnaires, amd biochemical and other diagnostic testing procedures. The survey covered 64 randomly selected geographical locations between 1976 and 1980, involving a multistage probability sample of all persons aged 6 months to 74 years. Detailed information on the sample design and operation of NHANES II have been described elsewhere.[10]

In the NHANES II survey, a cigarette smoker is defined as a person who has smoked at least 100 cigarettes and is currently a smoker (includes occasional smokers). Age-specific levels of risk associated with serum cholesterol are defined according to a National Institutes of Health Consensus Development Conference on "Lowering Blood Cholesterol to Prevent Heart Disease"[11]:

Age	Moderate risk	High risk
20-29	200-219 mg/dL	> 220 mg/dL
30-39	220-239 mg/dL	> 240 mg/dL
40+	240-259 mg/dL	> 260 mg/dL

The study for this report included 2,184 women aged 20 to 44 years. Women were excluded if they reported a history of myocardial infarction, stroke, or hardening of the arteries or were pregnant or lactating. The study population was divided into two groups, women currently taking OCs (n=504), and nonusers (no use during the past 6 months, n=1680). Users within the recent past (users in last 6 months but not currently using OCs, n=158) were eliminated from the analysis because of residual metabolic effects. Sampling survey weights were considered in calculating prevalence of smoking and serum cholesterol and blood pressure levels. Multiple regression was used to adjust for differences in discrete heart disease risk factors. For prevalence ratios, such as the percentage of high-risk women, adjustment for age was undertaken by the direct method of standardization to the total US female population aged 20 to 44 years.

RESULTS

In the WCCDS, smoking was more common among current OC users than among nonusers, while fewer current users reported a family history of heart disease. Nearly one third (32.8%) of the women taking the pill reported that they smoked, compared to 34.1% of the nonusers. Age, body mass index, and blood pressure were similar between the user and nonuser groups. In general, the three groups of women had approximately equal risk factors for heart disease, except for smoking and family history.

Progestin dose appeared to affect serum lipoprotein levels to the greatest degree, followed by smoking (Table 7-1). Both factors were associated with increased total and LDL cholesterols along with decreased HDL levels. The table suggests that a smoker using a low 0.4-mg norethindrone-dose OC can expect it to have less of an effect on HDL (1.6 mg/dL based on 0.4 x -4.0) than smoking's 2.4 mg/dL effect. Age and estrogen were associated with increased levels in all three lipoproteins, but only the increases for age were significant. The combined effect of smoking and a standard 1-mg norethindrone-containing OC is estimated to be -6 mg/dL, a substantial change of 10%.

In Table 7-2, mean lipid levels are presented for smoking, age, body mass index, and caffeine. For all pill users, total cholesterol level (206 mg/dL) is higher than for nonusers (196 mg/dL). The highest total cholesterol, and correspondingly lowest HDL cholesterol, are found among women using high-progestin, low-estrogen pills. The best HDL levels are found in women using the low norethindrone-containing formulations. Thus, the WCCDS data indicate that women who smoke and use low-estrogen, high-progestin pills may have poor heart disease risk profiles.

Table 7-1
Interactions Among Statistically Significant Cardiovascular Risk Factors for Women Participating in WCCDS

	Linear Coefficients				
				OC Dose	
Lipoprotein (mg/dL)	Smoker[1]	BMI[2]	AGE[3]	Estrogen	Progestin
Total cholesterol	0.5	.16	.54	.12	6.0
HDL cholesterol	-2.4	-.17	.36	.08	-4.0
LDL cholesterol	2.9	.32	.18	.04	10.0

1 Additional cholesterol effect in a smoker
2 Cholesterol effect per (lb/in^2).
3 For each year.

Table 7-2
Plasma Lipoprotein Concentrates Adjusted for Age, Body Mass Index, Cigarette and Caffeine Use According to User Group

			Serum Lipids (mg/dL)			
Exposure Group		No.	Total Choles-terol	HDL Choles-terol	LDL Choles-terol	Trigly-cerides
Never User		192	192.5	57.5	121.0	84.2
Past User		1123	198.4	59.7	124.2	86.7
Current User						
Estrogen (mg)	Norethindrone (mg)					
<.05	<1.5	106	201.8	60.0	121.1	123.8
<.05	>1.5	12	209.6	53.0	136.4	120.9
>.05	<1.5	72	208.3	63.3	123.5	129.0
>.05	>1.5	19	215.4	58.8	135.4	127.1

A more in-depth comparison of standard heart disease risk profiles for users and nonusers is possible from the NHANES II data. Means for standard heart disease risk factors were compared among OC users and nonusers representing the reproductive-age US female population, 1976-1980. Based on the design of the survey, the number of current users was estimated at 7 million, or 21% of women aged 20 to 44 years. As in the WCCDS cohort, OC users were likely to be significantly younger and less overweight than nonusers.

The mean total cholesterol of 205 mg/dL for OC users is approximately equal to that of the OC users in the WCCDS, while the value of 188 mg/dL demonstrated in the nonusers is somewhat lower than that for WCCDS control women (Table 7-3). The age-standardized prevalence of smoking, 44%, is higher in the OC users than the 35% in nonusers. Blood pressure is also slightly higher in the population-based sample of OC users compared to the nonusers. In the aggregate, it appears that OC users have a poorer aggregate cardiovascular risk profile compared to nonsmokers since mean smoking, total cholesterol, and blood pressure were all higher among OC users.

Table 7-4 presents the age-standardized percentages of women who have moderate-risk and high-risk cholesterol levels according to OC-user status. Standardization increases the proportion of high- and moderate-risk levels in the younger OC-user group. According to the Consensus Development Conference algorithm based on age and total cholesterol level, 38% of OC users are classified as high or moderate risk compared to 23% of nonusers, given that both groups have the age distribution of all US females aged 20 to 44 years. In consideration of all three risk factors, 61% of OC users had at least

Table 7-3
Mean Cardiovascular Risk Factors According to OC Use Adjusted for Age and Body Mass Index

Risk Factor	OC User (N = 504)	Non-User (N = 1680)	Significance of Difference
Serum Total Cholesterol (mg/dl)[1]	205	188	p = <.001
Blood Pressure (mmHg)[2]			
Systolic	116	113	p = <.001
Diastolic	74	73	p = .15
Smokers(%)[3]	44	36	p = .03

Source: Preventive Medicine[10]
[1] Adjusted for family history, other steroid use, smoking, and antihypertensive drug use.
[2] Standardized by direct method for age.
[3] Standardized by direct method for age.

Table 7-4
Cardiovascular Risk Profiles: Age-Adjusted Percentage of Females, 20-44, with Cardiovascular Risk Factors According to OC Use: United States 1976-1980

Risk Factor	OC User	Non-User
Smokers	43.9	35.4
Total Cholesterol		
Moderate Risk	15.7	11.3
High Risk	23.6	11.5
Blood Pressure		
> 140/90	8.6	8.0
> 160/95	3.2	3.5
Number of Risk Factors		
None	39.0	53.0
One	47.2	39.9
Two or Three	13.8	7.1

Source: Preventive Medicine

one heart disease risk factor compared to 47% of nonusers (Table 7-4). Among the risk factors, smoking appeared to be the most prevalent.

DISCUSSION

Cigarette smoking and OC use are independently associated with poorer cardiovascular risk profiles. National survey data indicate that while more than half of nonusers have no risk factors for heart disease, only 39% of OC users have completely normal cardiovascular risk profiles. A good portion of the disadvantage in OC users appeared to be related directly to an excess prevalence of smoking. Standardized estimates of smoking prevalence were 44% for OC users and 35% for nonusers, making smoking the most commonly abnormal component of the heart disease risk profile in young women.

Total cholesterol was the second most commonly abnormal component of the profile, with 39% of pill users and 22% of nonusers having an elevated total cholesterol value. The nature of the adverse effect on cholesterol was most effectively demonstrated from the WCCDS metabolic data set where progestin exposure affected cholesterol levels in a dose-response pattern. The HDL cholesterol decrease of 4 mg/dL and an increase in LDL cholesterol of 10 mg/dL per mg of the progestin were consistent with the estimate of an overall 6 mg/dL increase in total cholesterol for every 1 mg norethindrone used. In accordance with statistical model, smoking's effect is independent of but additive to norethindrone's adverse lipid effects. Smoking thus has a secondary indirect effect on the risk profile, adding an additional 3 mg/dL to LDL cholesterol and 0.5 mg/dL to total cholesterol. One can therefore estimate that smokers who use low dose (0.4 mg), standard dose (1 mg), and high dose (2 mg) norethindrone-containing OCs can expect 4 mg/dL, 6.5 mg/dL, and 10.5 mg/dL (or 16%) lower HDL levels than corresponding values for nonsmoking nonusers of the same age and body mass. Similarly, one can project total cholesterol to be higher by 5 mg/dL, 6.5 mg/dL, and 12.5 mg/dL among smoking OC users than among nonsmoking nonusers. In premenopausal women, HDL and total cholesterol effects of this magnitude are strongly predictive of future heart diseases.[5,6]

The maximum predicted cholesterol effect (12.5 mg/dL) is far lower than the observed 17 mg/dL total cholesterol difference between the national user and nonuser samples, suggesting a possible synergistic smoking-progestin effect. A statistically significant interaction could not be demonstrated, however. On the other hand, adjustments for substantial age differences between users and nonusers had some role in maximizing the mean cholesterol difference, and it is possible that most OC users of the late 1970s were using higher dose progestin formulations than women do today. The most likely explanation is that the excess of smoking among users accounts for a large portion of the measured cholesterol effect in users. This explanation is supported by the fact that the percentage of women with two or more risk factors is far lower than the combined percentages of women smokers and women with elevated cholesterol levels. Our data thus tend to reinforce the findings of one large propective study that shows smoking and elevated cholesterol to cluster in the same high-risk women.[12]

Our findings indicate that physicians will be confronted by many women who smoke, use the pill, and have poor cardiovascular risk profiles. Clinicians should be aware of the fact that an abnormal screening profile in a young OC user may be as likely to reflect the smoking effect as the physiologic or metabolic side effects of contraceptive progestins. Given the benefits associated with OC use, including reduced maternal mortality and lowered risk of endometrial and ovarian cancer, clinicians might be wise to consider smoking-cessation intervention as a first alternative to discontinuation of the pill.[1,13,14]

A rationale for smoking cessation among OC users is intuituve but can also be based on the following: (1) Clinical trials have demonstrated that smoking-cessation intervention can greatly improve one's prognosis for premature heart disease.[15] (2) There is a great amount of literature documenting smoking's role in the development of atherosclerotic lesions. (3) Several papers concerning the relationship between ever having smoked and lifetime risk of heart disease have been published.[16-18] The large body of literature on the adverse effects of smoking must be compared to the current lack of papers demonstrating an excess of progestin-related atherosclerotic disease in the population. Therefore, it is sensible to first consider smoking cessation and diet when considering ways to improve a woman's cardiovascular risk profile.[16]

Attempts to improve the heart disease risk profile of young OC users are important since progestin-induced lipoprotein effects may yet be shown to be related to increased or premature heart disease. In accordance with our results and the lipid hypothesis of atherogenesis, long-term lipid-related cardiocascular effects of the progestins, if they exist, will be latent and most evident in long-term, high progestin-dose OC users who smoke.[19,20] Using HDL-based myocardial infarction incidence projections derived from the Framingham study, the 16% decrease in HDL cholesterol for smoking, high progestin-dose OC users may result in a myocardial infarction risk in the range of 1.3 to 1.5.[2] Fortunately, the anticipated magnitude of this association is significantly lower in nonsmokers and in lower-dose users. Among groups of nonsmoking, low progestin-dose OC users who have suffered only 1.6 mg/dL (or 3.2%) HDL changes, relative risks are anticipated to be so low (1.1 or less) that they would be below the resolving power of epidemiologic studies.

SUMMARY

Any association between the pill and atherosclerotic heart disease will likely be confounded by cigarette smoking. Until the results of epidemiologic studies are known, physicians faced with an abnormal cardiovascular risk profile in a woman who smokes and who uses the pill should first consider smoking cessation intervention and diet.[15,17] If, after these interventions, a woman still displays a poor cardiovascular risk profile, the physician should can consider a lower-dose formulation or a brand of OC that contains a lower-potency progestin.[1] This may be superior to searching for an alternate method of birth control.

REFERENCES

1. Perlman JA, Russell-Briefel R, Ezzati T, et al: Oral glucose tolerance and the potency of contraceptive progestins. *J Chronic Dis* 1985;10:857-864.
2. Spellacy WN: A perspective on progestogens in oral contraceptives. *Am J Obstet Gynecol* 1982;142:717.
3. Wahl P, Walden C, Knopp R: Effect of estrogen/progestin potency on lipid/lipoprotein cholesterol. *N Engl J Med* 1983;308:862-867.
4. Abbott RD, Garrison RJ, Wilson PW, et al: Coronary heart disease risk: The importance of joint relationships among cholesterol levels in individual lipoprotein classes. *Prev Med* 1982;11:131-141.
5. Kannell WB, Castelli WP, Gordon T: Cholesterol in the prediction of atherosclerotic disease. *Ann Intern Med* 1979; 90:85-91.
6. Wilson PW, Garrison RJ, Castelli WP, et al: Prevalence of coronary heart disease in the Framingham Offspring Study: Role of lipoprotein cholesterols. *Am J Cardiology* 1980;46:649-654.
7. Ramcharan S, et al: The Walnut Creek Contraceptive Drug Study. Center for Population Research Monograph, vol 1, US Dept of Health, Education, and Welfare publication No. (NIH)74-562, 1974.
8. Ramcharan S, et al: The Walnut Creek Contraceptive Drug Study. Center for Population Research Monograph, vol 2, US Dept of Health, Education, and Welfare publication No. (NIH)76-563, 1976.
9. Ramcharan S, et al: The Walnut Creek Contraceptive Drug Study. Center for Population Research Monograph, vol 3, US Dept of Health, Education, and Welfare publication No. (NIH)81-564, 1981.
10. Russell-Briefel R, Ezzati T, Fulwood R, et al: Cardiovascular risk status and oral contraceptive use: United States 1976-1980. *Prev Med* 1986;15:352-363.
11. Lowering blood cholesterol to prevent heart disease. National Institutes of Health Consensus Development Conference Consensus Statement. *JAMA* 1985;253:14:2080-2090.
12. Simons LA, Simons J, Jones AS: The interactions of body weight, age, cigarette smoking, and hormone usage with blood pressure and plasma lipids in an Australian community. *Aust NZ J Med* 1984;14:215-221.
13. NIH Center for Population Research. *Report of the Center for Population Research.* Bethesda, Md. National Institute of Child and Human Development, 1985.
14. Ory H, Forrest J, Lincoln R: *Making Choices: Evaluating the Health Risks and Benefits of Birth Control Methods.* New York, Alan Guttmacher Institute, 1983.
15. Rabkin SW: Effect of cigarette smoking cessation on risk factors for coronary atherosclerosis: A controled clinical trial. *Atherosclerosis* 1984;53:173-184.

16. Brewer HB, Sprecher DL, Gregg RE, et al: Risk factors for the development of premature cardiovascular disease. *Adv Exp Med Biol* 1985;183:27-36.
17. Heller RF, Chinn S, Redoe HD, et al: How well can we predict coronary heart disease? Findings in the United Kingdom heart disease prevention project. *Br Med J Clin Res* 1984;288:1409-1411.
18. Holme I, Solberg LA, Weissfeld L, et al: Coronary risk factors and their pathway of action through coronary raised lesions, coronary stenoses and coronary death. Multivariate statistical analysis of an autopsy series: The Oslo Study. *Am J Cardiol* 1985,55.40-47.
19. Ross R, Faggiotto A, Bowen-Pope D, et al: The role of endothelial injury and platelet and macrophage interactions in atherosclerosis. *Circulation* 1984;70:1177-1182.
20. Wilson PWF, Garrison RJ, Abbott RD, et al: Factors associated with lipoprotein cholesterol levels: The Framingham study. *Artheriosclerosis* 1983;3(3):273-281.

8 *Smoking, Oral Contraceptives, and Cardiovascular Disease: An International Perspective*

Susan Holck, Ramon Aznar, Rebecca Wang, Lothar Heinemann, Michael Marmot, M. Shipley

---

Numerous studies from North America and Western Europe demonstrate an increased risk of cardiovascular disease among women using combined oral contraceptives (OC).[1,2] Specifically, OCs containing at least 50 ug of estrogen increase the risk of venous thromboembolic disease, myocardial infarction, and stroke. In the United States and the United Kingdom, where most of the studies have been conducted, the increased risk of cardiovascular disease attributable to OC use appears to be concentrated among women 35 years or older and among women who smoke.

Although OCs are recognized as increasing the risk of cardiovascular disease, particularly among smokers, data on this issue are lacking in two important areas. First, little information is available on cardiovascular effects of the commonly used "low dose" preparations containing 30 or 35 µg of ethinyl estradiol. Second, little information exists on the association among OCs, smoking, and cardiovascular disease risk in countries outside North America and Western Europe.

Cardiovascular risk factors and disease vary widely throughout the world, and specific risk factors contribute differently to cardiovascular disease risk in different populations. For example, in black populations in the Caribbean, the prevalence of hypertension is high, but coronary heart disease is rare.[3] The effect of OCs or smoking on cardiovascular disease risk may also vary among populations.

Two case-control studies have been published on OC use and cardiovascular risk. In 1984, Aznar and Lara published a report of a hospital-based case-control study of cardiovascular disease and OC use in Mexico.[4] The estimated relative risk (RR) of cardiovascular disease was 1.4 among OC users (P-value $<.05$). The increased risk was confined primarily to women aged 40 to 44 years, among whom the estimated RR was 3.6. The RR of cardiovascular disease among current smokers was also 1.4 ($P <.01$). There was no evidence of any overall interaction between OC use and smoking with respect to cardiovascular disease risk. The report does not mention whether women with a previous history of cardiovascular disease were included.

The association between mortality from cardiovascular disease and OC use was examined in a study by Chow et al from Taiwan.[5] Unfortunately, women who had reportedly used OCs at the time of their deaths were grouped with women who had previously used OCs at any time to make up the exposed groups. Thus it was not possible to calculate the risk of cardiovascular disease mortality among current OC users. This could account for the lack of any association in this study between OC use and cardiovascular disease mortality.

One other limited study of the incidence of deep vein thrombosis and OC use among Chinese women was published by Tso et al.[6] Among 43 OC users, two had evidence of venous thrombosis; among the 81 nonusers, none had evidence of venous thrombosis. There was no mention of smoking in the report.

These three studies provide only limited information on OC use, smoking, and cardiovascular disease risk, and all three suffer from methodologic problems. The study by Aznar and Lara[4] does suggest that the risk of cardiovascular disease may be increased by OC use and smoking among populations outside the United States and Europe. Because of the lack of information on cardiovascular disease risk and smoking and oral contraceptive use in developing countries, in 1979 the World Health Organization initiated a case-control study of cardiovascular disease in Hong Kong and Mexico. The same protocol was later used for a study in the German Democratic Republic.

METHODS

Cases were selected from married women aged 20 to 44 years admitted to the hospital with a diagnosis of cardiovascular disease. Three controls were selected for each case from women admitted with diagnoses thought not to be related to contraceptive use and without a previous history of cardiovascular disease. Controls were matched to cases by age within 5-year age groups and by parity (parous, non-parous). The subjects were interviewed about their contraceptive and smoking histories, as well as other known risk factors for cardiovascular disease.

Cases of rheumatic heart disease were excluded from analysis because the confounding with pre-existing heart disease and OC use made the results uninterpretable. Similarly, all cases that were not newly diagnosed were excluded from the analyses. Thus, we were able to analyze preliminary data on 65 cases from Mexico, 141 from Hong Kong, and 77 from the German Democratic Republic. Data collection was still ongoing in Mexico and the German Democratic Republic at the time of these analyses; the final report will include additional subjects from these two centers.

RESULTS

Smoking was more common among cases than controls in all three centers. In Mexico, 28% of cases and 23% of controls were current smokers; in Hong Kong, 9% of cases and 4% of controls; and in the German Democratic Republic, 29% of cases and 23% of controls (Table 8-1). The overall relative risk of cardiovascular disease among current smokers (relative to nonsmokers) was 1.4 in Mexico and the German Democratic Republic and 2.2 in Hong Kong and 2.0, 1.1, and 1.5 respectively among former smokers. Data on the association between OC use and cardiovascular disease are not yet available.

Table 8-1
Subjects in WHO Collaborative Study of Cardiovascular Disease and Oral Contraceptives and Percent Former Smokers and Current Smokers, by Center

Center	Cases*			Controls		
	No.	Former Smokers(%)	Current Smokers(%)	No.	Former Smokers(%)	Current Smokers(%)
Mexico	65	12.3	27.7	126	7.1	23.0
Hong Kong	141	2.1	9.2	391	1.5	4.3
German Democratic Republic	77	9.1	28.6	166	9.0	22.9

* Includes all newly diagnosed cases of nonrheumatic heart disease, stroke, and pulmonary embolus or deep venous thrombosis.

Table 8-2
Percent of Controls Who Used Contraception in Previous Month, by Method Used Among Never- and Current Smokers, by Center, WHO Collaborative Study

Most recent method used in previous month	Mexico		Hong Kong		German Democratic Republic	
	Never smokers(%) n=391	Current smokers(%) n=134	Never smokers(%) n=1177	Current smokers(%) n=52	Never smokers(%) n=708	Curre smoke n=
Oral Contraceptives	13.0	13.4	9.3	25.0	31.2	42
Injectables	4.6	3.7	2.1	1.9	1.3	0.
IUD	22.8	18.7	4.7	1.9	6.8	6.
Sterilized*	27.6	28.4	27.2	40.4	0.1	0.
Other method	22.0	23.9	37.1	15.3	24.9	19.

* subject or husband sterilized

Among the controls, OC use was more prevalent among smokers than among nonsmokers in all three centers, although the difference was minimal in Mexico (Table 8-2). These preliminary analyses suggest that smoking may increase the risk of cardiovascular disease in Mexico (confirming the report of Aznar and Lara), Hong Kong, and the German Democratic Republic. If OCs also increase the risk of cardiovascular disease, the findings of a higher proportion of OC users among women who smoke is of potential concern.

DISCUSSION

Little information is available from developing countries on the cardiovascular disease risk among women who use OCs and/or smoke. Nor do we know the extent to which OC use or smoking contributes to cardiovascular disease in these countries. However, we do know that OC use is increasing in many developing countries and that up to one fourth of married women of reproductive age report using OCs in Thailand, parts of Brazil, Costa Rica, and some Caribbean countries.[7] Although the prevalence of smoking is still low among women in many developing countries, in some countries smoking is becoming increasingly common among women; more than one fourth of women of reproductive age smoke in such countries as Mexico, Argentina, Brazil, Chile, Colombia and Venezuela.[8] Furthermore, mortality from cardiovascular disease appears to increase with urbanization.[9] Thus, the incidence of cardiovascular disease can be expected to increase in developing countries along with socioeconomic development.

In countries where smoking prevalence is still low among women and where morbidity and mortality from cardiovascular disease is minimal, use of OCs probably contribute little cardiovascular disease risk. However, in the countries where as many as one fourth of the women smoke and where the incidence of cardiovascular disease is not minimal, we need information on both the effect of OC use and smoking on cardiovascular disease risk as well as the extent of smoking by OC users. Until we have this information, it is prudent to assume that OC use and smoking do increase the risk of cardiovascular disease in these countries. Therefore, women in developing countries must be encouraged not to smoke, especially those who are older and use oral contraceptives.

REFERENCES

1. Stadel BV: Oral contraceptives and cardiovascular disease. *N Engl J Med* 1981;305:612-618.
2. Stadel BV: Oral contraceptives and cardiovascular disease. *N Engl J Med* 1981;305:672-677.
3. Watkins LO: Coronary heart disease and coronary risk factors in black populations in underdeveloped countries: The case for primordial prevention. *Am Heart J* 1984;108: 850-862.
4. Aznar-Ramos R, Lara-Ricalde R: En fermedades cardiovasculares y anticoncepcion oral. Estudio de casos y controles. *Gac Med Mex* 1984;120:117-126.
5. Chow LP, Lin CC, Keyuan-Larijan E, et al: Oral contraceptives and mortality from circulatory system diseases: an epidemiologic study in Taiwan. *Int J Gynaecol Obstet* 1983;21:297-304.
6. Tso SC. Wong V, Chan V, et al: Deep vein thrombosis and changes in coagulation and fibrinolysis after gynaecological operations in Chinese: The effect of oral contraceptives and malignant disease. *Br J Haematol* 1980;46:603-612.
7. Population Information Program: Oral contraceptives in the 80s. Population Reports, Series A, No 6, Baltimore, The Johns Hopkins University, 1982.
8. WHO International Clearinghouse on Smoking and Health: Information, WHO documents WHO/SMO/83.1.
9. Tyroler HA, Cassel J: Health consequences of culture changes. II. The effect of urbanization on coronary heart mortality in rural residents. *J Chron Dis* 1964;17:167-177.

9 *Cigarette Smoking and Primary Tubal Infertility*

Janet Daling, Noel Weiss, Leon Spadoni, Donald E. Moore, Lynda Voigt

The effects of cigarette smoking on the performance of the female reproductive system have not been extensively studied.[1,2] Experimental evidence suggests that cigarette smoke can alter hypothalamic-pituitary interrelationships by stimulating growth hormone, cortisol, vasopressin, and oxytocin release and inhibiting luteinizing hormone and prolactin release.[3-6] These changes may alter the hormonal interrelationships necessary for successful reproduction. Studies in rodents, humans, and nonhuman primates also suggest that cigarette smoke reduces the motility of the female reproductive tract and may impair implantation of the embryo.[7-11] As part of a population-based, case-control study of infertility in relation to contraceptive practices, we have compared the smoking experience of women seeking treatment for infertility with that of fertile women.

METHODS

We sought to identify and interview all 20- to 39-year-old female residents of King County, Washington, whose first medical evaluation for infertility occurred during 1979-1981. All physicians in the county who performed such evaluations were contacted, and 89.5% agreed to cooperate in the study.

The focus of the study is on women with primary infertility (ie, those who have never conceived despite unprotected intercourse for at least 1 year) in whom a tubal condition was believed to be responsible. This judgment, made by the patient's physician, was based on either an abnormal hysterosalpingogram (HSG) or a tubal abnormality identified during surgery. If both HSG and surgery were performed but produced conflicting diagnoses, the surgical diagnosis was used. Seventy-two percent of the cases had undergone surgery.

We used Washington State Vital Records to identify married King County residents who gave birth during the calendar year following the one in which the case started trying to become pregnant. From the information contained in the birth record, each control was matched to a case by race, census tract of residence, and age (within 5-year groups) and was included only if she had never previously been pregnant.

A structured interview was conducted by a trained female interviewer in the subject's home. It included questions on reproductive, contraceptive, medical, and sexual histories, personal hygiene, demographic characteristics, and the use of "social" drugs, tobacco and alcohol, by both the woman and her husband. From women who had smoked cigarettes at some time in their lives, we also obtained information on the number of cigarettes they usually smoked per day, the age at which they began smoking, and if they quit smoking, the age at which they quit. We also asked the women if they were smokers at the "reference date," ie, the time at which the infertile subjects began to attempt to conceive.

The percentage of infertile subjects who were interviewed, 78.3%, was somewhat higher than that for controls, 72.7%, because a larger proportion of controls than cases had moved from the area or were lost to follow-up. (The controls were known only to be residents at some time between 1970-1980, coinciding with the time the cases started trying to become pregnant.) Lost to follow-up were 7.9% of cases and 20.5% of controls; 11.9% of cases and 6.8% of controls refused an interview. The percentage of women with primary tubal infertility who responded is not known, since it was not possible to review the charts and thus obtain a diagnosis for women who were not interviewed.

Of the 552 women with primary infertility whom we interviewed, 175 had a diagnosis of tubal infertility. For one of these cases, we were unable to locate a matched control, and in four other pairs data on exposure information of interest were missing. Thus, 170 matched pairs were available for the study. We analyzed the data obtained on them by a conditional logistic regression technique[12] for matched data, which estimates the odds ratio. Because the relative risk is estimated accurately by the odds ratio and because relative risk has greater intuitive meaning, we have used that term in this paper. The interview responses that were used in the analysis relate to events prior to the reference date.

RESULTS

Although cases and controls were demographically quite similar, the cases did tend to report a higher family income. On the average, the cases had more marriages and sexual partners than did controls. A history of IUD use was more commonly reported by the women with tubal infertility (33%) than by controls (14%).

In evaluating the possible difference between cases and controls with respect to smoking, we adjusted for the effects of the following confounding variables by including them in a conditional logistic regression model: IUD use—ever, never; number of sexual partners during their lives—<5, 5-9, 10-14, 15+; and annual family income—<$15,000, $15,000-$30,000, >$30,000. Variables that were assessed but did not influence the risk estimates associated with cigarette smoking included use of other methods of contraception (oral contraceptives, condoms, barrier methods); education; religion; "social" drug use; cigarette smoking by the husband; appendectomy; pelvic surgery; age at first intercourse; history of genital herpes; history of gonorrhea; and the use of douches.

A higher percentage of the cases (39%) than controls (16%) were smokers at the time they started trying to conceive (relative risk [RR] = 2.7; 95% confidence interval [CI] = 1.4-5.3). Former smokers, however, had little increase in risk compared with women who had never smoked (relative risk 1.1, CI = 0.5-2.5).

Among current smokers, women who had over 5 pack-years of exposure had 4.2 times the risk of tubal infertility of women who had never smoked (Table 9-1); the excess risk among other smokers was smaller (RR = 1.6) and could have occurred by chance. The size of the smoking/infertility association also varied according to the age at which a woman began smoking and according to the usual amount smoked, but to a lesser degree. No increase in risk was observed for former smokers with any of these smoking patterns. The lack of association with former smoking was present no matter how recently a woman had stopped (in the broad categories of ≤5 years ago and >5 years ago).

Women who had used certain types of IUDs were at increased risk of primary tubal infertility.[13] Compared with women who never smoked and had never used an IUD, the risk of tubal infertility in women smokers who had never used an IUD was 2.6 (95% CI = 1.2-5.6) (Table 9-2). Among women who used both an IUD and smoked, this relative risk was 6.7 (95% CI = 1.4-32.2), a value that suggests roughly a multiplicative effect of the two exposures on risk. In our previous analysis,[13] we found that the risks associated with the various types of IUDs were quite different. Women who had used only a copper IUD were at very little, if any, increased risk of tubal infertility. Among women who had used only copper IUDs, the risk among current smokers was only 40% higher than that of nonsmokers who used these IUDs. However, the number of subjects in these two categories (14 cases and eight controls) greatly limits any conclusion that can be made from this observation. Similarly, the risk of tubal infertility in women smokers with more than five sexual partners during their lifetimes appeared to be roughly the product of the relative risks associated with each exposure alone (Table 9-3).

DISCUSSION

One limitation of our study is that, although we came close to indentifying all women in a defined population whose infertility came to medical attention, we could not identify the infertile women who did not seek care. These women could represent a substantial proportion of those who are infertile, since the cost of an infertility workup is high and rarely covered by insurance. No such selectivity took place in the identification of our control subjects. Thus, if cigarette smoking was particularly common in the subgroup of infertile women who came to medical attention, the excess risks

Table 9-1
Patterns of Cigarette Smoking Among Women with Primary Tubal Infertility and Controls

Current Smokers

Characteristics	Cases (N=67) No.	Cases %	Controls (N=27) No.	Controls %	Relative Risk*	95% Confidence Interval
Age started smoking						
≤ 16 yr	31	18.2	10	5.9	4.3	1.6-11.1
> 16 yr	36	21.2	17	10.0	2.2	0.9- 5.1
Usual No. of cigarettes per day						
≤ 1/2 Pack	25	14.7	11	6.6	2.0	0.7- 5.3
> 1/2 Pack	42	24.7	16	9.4	3.2	1.4- 7.0
Pack-years of smoking+						
≤ 5	31	18.2	17	11.0	1.6	0.7- 3.8
> 5	36	21.2	10	5.9	4.2	1.8-10.2

Former Smokers

Characteristics	Cases (N=24) No.	Cases %	Controls (N=28) No.	Controls %	Relative Risk*	95% Confidence Interval
Age started smoking						
≤ 16 yr	6	3.5	9	5.3	0.6	0.1- 2.6
> 16 yr	18	10.6	19	11.2	1.4	0.6- 3.6
Usual No. of cigarettes per day						
≤ 1/2 pack	13	7.6	14	8.3	1.2	0.4- 3.3
> 1/2 pack	11	6.5	14	8.3	1.1	0.4- 3.3
Pack-years of Smoking+						
≤ 5	15	8.8	21	12.4	0.9	0.3-2.1
> 5	9	5.3	7	4.1	2.0	0.6-7.4
Time since stopping smoking						
≤ 5 yr	16	9.4	16	9.4	1.4	0.7- 3.0
> 5 yr	8	4.7	12	7.1	0.9	0.4- 2.4

* Risk relative to that of women who never smoked, adjusted for IUD use, income, and lifetime number of sexual partners.
\+ Pack-Year = Average packs per day times years smoked.

Table 9-2
Relation of Cigarette Smoking to the Risk of Primary Tubal Infertility According to IUD Use

Smoking Status	IUD Use	No. Cases	No. Cases	Relative Risk*	95% Confidence Interval
Never Smoked	Never	52	98	1.0	
Current Smoker	Never	48	25	2.6	1.2- 5.6
Never Smoked	Ever	27	17	2.3	1.0- 5.3
Current Smoker	Ever	19	2	6.7	1.4-32.2

* Risk relative to that of women who never smoked and never used and IUD, adjusted for income and number of sexual partners.

associated with smoking that we estimated may be falsely elevated. Nonetheless, we believe that this potential bias is unlikely to have occurred, for in our study there was no association between smoking and primary infertility due to other mechanisms, eg, endometriosis or ovulatory or cervical abnormalities.

Another limitation arises from the possibility that both smoking and tubal infertility are related to a factor that we could not adequately assess, eg, a woman's exposure to sexually transmitted infections that could cause tubal damage. Our measures of past infections were not at all precise (subject recall of clinical infections, number of sexual partners), and so some confounding could well have remained even after the data were adjusted for these variables.

Table 9-3
Relation of Cigarette Smoking to the Risk of Primary Tubal Infertility According to Lifetime Number of Sexual Partners

Smoking Status	Sexual Partners	No. Cases	No. Cases	Relative Risk*	95% Confidence Interval
Never Smoked	1-4	57	96	1.0	
Current Smoker	1-4	28	18	2.7	1.2- 6.2
Never Smoked	≥ 5	22	19	1.6	0.7- 3.6
Current Smoker	≥ 5	39	9	5.2	2.1-12.5

* Risk relative to women who never smoked and who had 1-4 sexual partners, adjusted for income and IUD use.

Finally, our analysis was restricted to nulligravid women, and any generalizations made from our results should be similarly restricted.

In two previous cohort studies of women attempting to conceive, a higher rate of failure was found in cigarette smokers. Howe et al[14] monitored women who had stopped contraception to become pregnant. They found a consistent and highly significant trend of decreasing fertility with increasing number of cigarettes smoked per day. Five years after stopping contraception, 10.7% of heavy smokers but only 4% of nonsmokers had not become pregnant. As in our study, ex-smokers did not show any evidence of decreased fertility compared with lifetime nonsmokers. Baird and Wilcox[15] looked at delay in conception in 678 women who became pregnant. Smokers were 3.4 times more likely than nonsmokers to have taken longer than a year to conceive. Olsen et al[16] in their case-control study, found a higher proportion of cases of both primary and secondary infertility to be smokers than controls. The authors stated that "significantly" more women with obstructed fallopian tubes were smokers than were women with other types of infertility, but they did not present any supporting data. Cramer et al[17] found that 56.7% of women with tubal infertility had ever smoked compared with 45.6% of fertile controls; they found no differences in the smoking histories of women with other types of infertility and those of the controls. We found that women who smoked cigarettes were at increased risk of primary tubal infertility, but not of other types of primary infertility. For instance, 20.1% of women who were found to have primary ovulatory dysfunction as the only explanation for their infertility were smokers, compared with 21.5% of their controls (RR = 0.7, 95% CI = 0.4-1.3). The relative risks associated with smoking for other types of infertility were similarly close to 1.0.

On the whole, the data suggest that cigarette smoking predisposes a woman to tubal infertility. We can only speculate as to the reasons for this. Smoking may alter a woman's response to sexually transmitted infections: humoral and cellular immunity are reduced by exposure to cigarette smoking.[18-23] Drac and Kopecny[11] found that smokers were more likely to have vaginal infections with Trichomonas, adnexal (ovary and fallopian tube) inflammation, and abnormal hysterosalpingograms. Nicotine also might have a toxic effect on the epithelium, facilitating the entry of pathogens.[24]

Our results need to be confirmed and extended. Future epidemiologic studies should focus on specific types of infertility and include serologic tests for sexually transmitted diseases. In addition, laboratory studies are needed to determine the effect of cigarette smoking on tubal pathology.

REFERENCES

1. Sterling TD, Kobayashi D: A critical review of reports on the effect of smoking on sex and fertility. *J Sex Res* 1975;11:201-217.
2. Weathersbee PS: Nicotine and its influence on the female reproductive system. *J Reprod Med* 1980;25:243-250.

3. Bisset GY, Feldberg W, Guerzenstein PG, et al.: Vasopressin release by nicotine: the site of action. *Br J Pharmacol* 1975;54:463-474.
4. Johnson LY, Vaughn MK, Reiter RJ, et al.: The effects of arginine vasotocin on pregnant mare's serum-induced ovulation in the immature female rat. *Acta Endocrinol* 1978;87:367-376.
5. Yamashita K, Mieno M, Yamashita ER: Suppression of the luteinizing hormone releasing effect of luteinizing hormone releasing hormone by arginine-vasotocin. *J Endocrinol* 1979;81:103-108.
6. McLean BK, Rubel A, Nikitovitch-Winer MB: The differential effects of exposure to tobacco smoke on the secretion of luteinizing hormone and prolactin in the proestrous rat. *Endocrinology* 1977;100:1566-1570.
7. Neri A, Eckerling B: Influence of smoking and adrenaline (epinephrine) on the uterotubal insufflation test (Rubin test). *Fertil Steril* 1969;20:818-828
8. Neri A, Marcus SL: Effect of nicotine on the motility of the oviducts in the rhesus monkey: A preliminary report. *J Reprod Fertil* 1972;31:91-97.
9. Ruckebusch Y: Relationship between the electrical activity of the oviduct and uterus of the rabbit in vivo. *J Reprod Fertil* 1975;45:73-82.
10. Yoshinaga K, Rice K, Krenn J, et al: Effects of nicotine on early pregnancy in the rat. *Biol Reprod* 1979;20:294-303.
11. Drac P, Kopecny J: Sterilitat bei Raucherinnen and Nichtraucherinnen. *Zentralbl Gynakol* 1970;27:865-866.
12. Breslow NE, Day NE: Statistical methods in cancer research: The analysis of case-control studies. *IARC Sci Publ* 1980;1: No. 32.
13. Daling JR, Weiss NS, Metch BJ, et al: Primary tubal infertility in relation to the use of an intrauterine device. *N Engl J Med* 1985;312:937-941.
14. Howe G, Westhoff C, Vessey M, et al: Effects of age, cigarette smoking, and other factors on fertility: findings in a large prospective study. *Br Med J* 1985;290:1697-1700.
15. Baird DD, Wilcox AJ: Cigarette smoking associated with delayed conception. *JAMA* 1985;20:2979-2983.
16. Olsen J, Rachootin P, Schiodt AV, et al: Tobacco use, alcohol consumption and infertility. *Int J Epidemiol* 1983;2:179-184.
17. Cramer DW, Schiff I, Schoenbaum SC, et al: Tubal infertility and the intrauterine device. *N Engl J Med* 1985;312:941-947.
18. Onari K, Seyama A, Inamitzu T, et al: Immunological study on cigarette smokers. Part 1. Serum protein pattern in smokers. *Hiroshima J Med Sci* 1978;27:113-118.
19. Onari K, Sadamoto K, Takaishi M, et al: Immunological studies on cigarette smokers. Part 1. Cell mediated immunity in cigarette smokers and the influence of the water-soluble fraction of cigarette smoke on the immunity of mice. *Hiroshima J Med Sci* 1980;29:29-35.
20. Winkel P, Statland BE: The acute effect of cigarette smoking on the concentrations of blood leukocyte types in healthy young women. *Am J Clin Pathol* 1981;75:781-785.
21. Anderson P, Pederson OF, Bach B, et al: Serum antibodies and immunoglobulins in smokers and nonsmokers. *Clin Exp Immunol* 1982;47:467-473.
22. Hersey P, Prendergast D, Edwards A: Effects of cigarette smoking on the immune system. Follow-up studies in normal subjects after cessation of smoking. *Med J Aust* 1983;2:425-429.
23. Burton RC: Smoking, immunity, and cancer. *Med J Aust* 1983;2:411-412.
24. Singer A, Walker PG, McCance DJ: Genital wart virus infections: nuisance or potentially lethal? *Br Med J* 1984;288:735-736.

10 *The Effect of Smoking on Reproductive Ability and Reproductive Lifespan*

Donald R. Mattison
Peter J. Thomford

This review focuses on three topics: first, clinical evidence and animal models which suggest that women who smoke cigarettes are less readily able to become pregnant and have a shorter reproductive life span than women who do not smoke; second, smoking's effect on sex steroid metabolism; finally, a mathematical model is described which explores how reproductive toxins such as cigarette smoke alter the reproductive life-span. The effect of altered oocyte number or rate of atresia on age of menopause will be evaluated with this model.

FECUNDITY

In the female, as in the male, successful reproduction requires a series of integrated events.[1-3] In the human female, the major controlling organ is the ovary, which is responsible for gamete production and maturation as well as steroid hormone production and secretion.[4] Most of the available evidence suggests that the ovary is vulnerable to insult by one or more toxins contained in cigarette smoke[5] as well as other xenobiotics.[6]

Hammond found that abnormal vaginal bleeding, a measure of abnormal hypothalamic-pituitary-ovarian function, increases with increasing cigarette consumption.[7] At the time this study was conducted, abnormal vaginal bleeding was a major indication for hysterectomy. He also hypothesized that if smoking does interfere with this endocrine balance to cause abnormal bleeding, that this will result in a greater likelihood of hysterectomy. He found that nonsmokers had the lowest hysterectomy rate, followed by former smokers, light smokers, and heavy smokers. He also found that among women who had hysterectomies, the proportion who had irregular bleeding was strongly associated with smoking: 14.8% of nonsmokers had irregular menses prior to surgery, compared with 13.2% of exsmokers, 16.1% of women smoking fewer than 20 cigarettes per day, and 16.4% of women smoking more than 20 cigarettes per day.

In 1968, Tokuhata explored the effects of smoking on fertility in a case-control survey of women dying of breast cancer.[8] Infertility, defined as no pregnancy by the end of a woman's reproductive life, was 12.4% among white nonsmokers and 18.8% among nonwhite nonsmokers. Among smokers, however, the respective proportions were 16.6% and 28.2%. This suggests that either cigarettes contain some substance deleterious to reproduction or a lifestyle factor associated with cigarettes was responsible for the infertility.

Recent studies also demonstrate that women who smoke have a variety of menstrual cycle abnormalities and impaired ability to conceive and to bear children.[5,9-11] Baird and Wilcox counted the number of menstrual cycles from cessation of contraception to pregnancy and found that smokers had a lower cumulative percent pregnancy rate than nonsmokers.[9] During the first 18 cycles in particular, smokers are strikingly less likely to become pregnant than nonsmokers. Strong as these effects are, they may actually underestimate the true strength that smoking has, since the study was biased against demonstrating an adverse effect of smoking by its requirement that all women included must have become pregnant within 2 years of cessation of contraception. Howe et al examined the same question by evaluating the time required to deliver an infant after stopping contraception (Figure 10-1).[10] Fifty-nine percent of nonsmokers had delivered by 12 months after stopping contraception, while 56.2% of women smoking 11-15 cigarettes, and 49.1% of women smoking more than 21 cigarettes per day had. This dose-dependent effect of cigarette smoking on fertility persisted over the 60 months of observation.

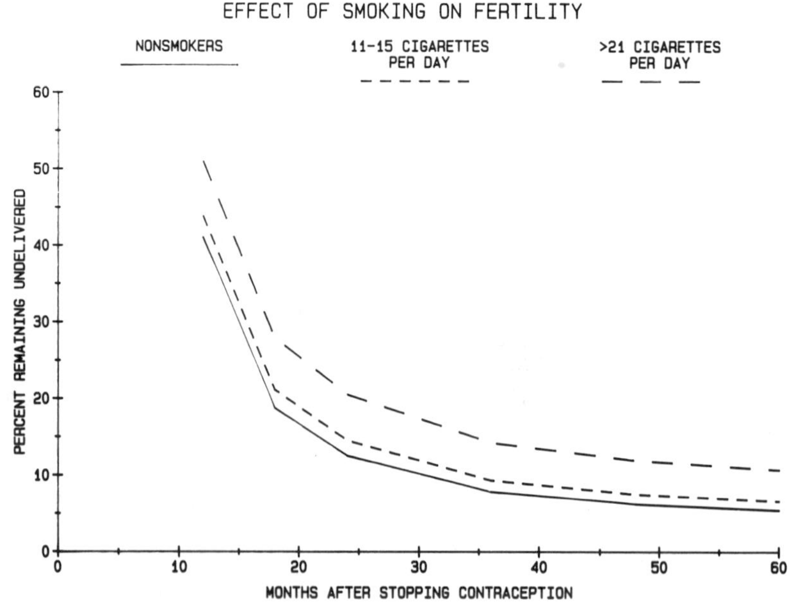

Figure 10-1 Effect of smoking on fertility.

AGE AT MENOPAUSE

Women who smoke undergo earlier menopause than do nonsmokers,[5,12] and two studies suggest the reduction in age is a function of the degree of smoking.[13,14] At most ages, smokers were more likely to be menopausal than nonsmokers (Figure 10-2). Within each age group, greater cigarette consumption increased the likelihood of being menopausal. Similar cigarette dose dependent decreases in age at menopause were demonstrated by Jick et al in 1977.[14] In that study, women who smoked approximately half a pack of cigarettes per day had a median age of menopause about a year younger than nonsmokers. Women smoking a pack or more per day had a mean age of menopause approximately 2 years younger.

BENZO(A)PYRENE AND MURINE FECUNDITY

We began a series of experiments to define the reproductive effects of benzo(a)pyrene and its metabolites. In the first experiment, mice treated with increasing doses of benzo(a)pyrene showed progressively lower numbers of pups produced.[15] The data suggested that benzo(a)pyrene, one component of the tar fraction in cigarette smoke, is a potent reproductive toxin in animals, decreasing fertility in a dose-dependent fashion. A subsequent experiment ex-

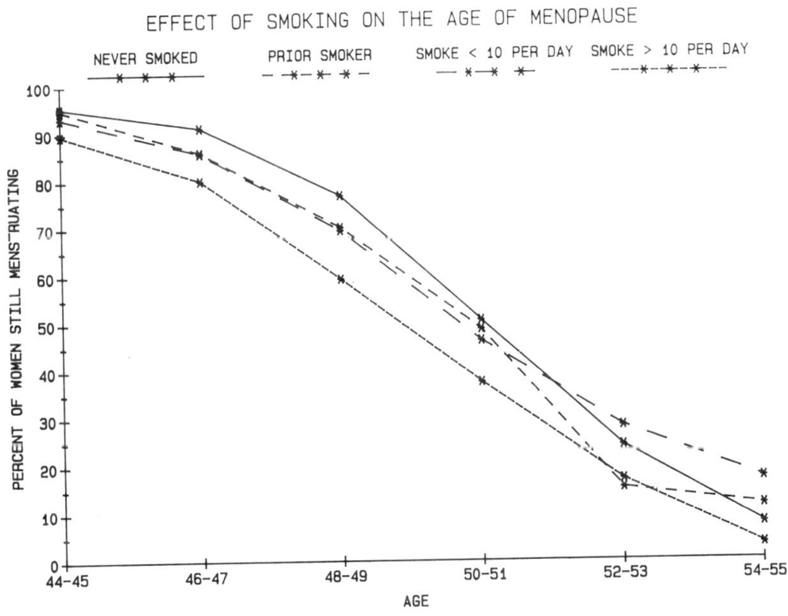

Figure 10-2 Effect of smoking on age of menopause.

amined the effect of lower doses (1-50 mg/kg) and found that increasing the dose increased the interval between births (Mattison DR, MD; Silbergeld E, PhD; Malley K, MS, 1984, unpublished data). Later experiments consisted of counting corpora lutea of mice treated with benzo(a)pyrene.[16] The number of corpora lutea reflect the number of oocytes produced. The data suggest that the decrease in number of corpora lutea recovers over a 3- to 4-week period after a single-dose treatment. This decrease in ovulatory rate may account for the decreases in fertility and increased time required to attain pregnancy observed in women smokers.

BENZO(A)PYRENE AND MURINE OOCYTE DESTRUCTION

In an experiment designed to examine the influence of benzo(a)pyrene on number of oocytes, mice treated intraperitoneally with doses between 5 and 500 mg/kg, experienced a clear dose-dependent decrease in oocyte number. The reproductive lifespan of the mice was shortened over control subjects, with the highest doses having the shortest reproductive lives. In the human female, the age of menopause reflects the cessation of reproductive competence. A cigarette dose-dependent decrease in the age of menopause appears analogous to the experimental decrease in reproductive life-span following treatment with benzo(a)pyrene, a component of cigarette smoke.

SMOKING AND HORMONE METABOLISM

Reduced levels of circulating estrogens may be a factor in mediating smoking-related impairment in reproduction. Drugs and naturally occurring steroids such as estrogen, progesterone, and testosterone are metabolized by NADPH-dependent mixed function oxidase system found in the liver. The multiplicity and wide tissue distribution of these mixed function oxidase enzymes makes their role in steroid metabolism difficult to interpret. Many xenobiotics appear to increase the hepatic clearance of steroids and thus decrease their blood levels. What is less clear is the effect that these drugs have on other tissues. What is also not clear is which forms of P-450 are induced by which chemicals and which forms are responsible for metabolizing steroids. Smoking may affect production of ovarian steroids by altering steroid-producing cytochrome P-450 enzymes.[19]

MacMahon et al showed that urinary estrogens are reduced in smoking women during the luteal phase but not during the follicular phase,[20] consistent with the theory that ovarian production and/or urinary excretion of estrogen is impaired by smoking. This study unfortunately did not include measurements to differentiate between the two effects.

Studies suggest a major impact of smoking on the hypothalamic pituitary-gonad-liver axis, possibly mediated by changes in gonadal and hepatic steroid metabolism.[21] Whether these effects are due to changes in P-450-dependent metabolism or effects on mitochondrial conversion of cholesterol to pregnenolone is a topic for further investigation.

A MATHEMATICAL MODEL OF MENOPAUSE

In integrating the results of studies summarized so far, it is apparent that one mechanism by which smoking might shorten a woman's reproductive life is by reducing the number of oocytes and thus hastening menopause. The decrease in number of oocytes and its relationship to onset of menopause is presented in Figure 10-3. This in turn has implications for the onset of other diseases, such as endometrial cancer, which is reduced in smokers, and breast cancer, which is reduced in women with early menopause.

Human data suggest that smoking one pack of cigarettes per day decreases the age of menopause by 2 years. The data of Block[24] permit estimation of the number of oocytes which must be destroyed if this is the case. Based on counting the number of oocytes among women who died traumatic deaths, the number of oocytes at any given age is

$$\text{No. oocytes (a)} = 901\ e\text{-}0.127a$$

where a=age (Figure 10-3, top panel). The center panel illustrates how changing the number of oocytes present at birth changes the age of menopause; for example, to produce premature ovarian failure and menopause at age 35, a woman would have to born with 20% of the normal number of oocytes. Premature menopause can also result in a woman born with a normal number of oocytes but who undergoes increased rates of atresia, such as might be expected from cigarettes (panel C). For example, menopause at age 35 requires only a 1.5-fold increase in the rate of atresia. If smoking simply destroys oocytes, destruction of about 20% of oocytes would be necessary to decrease the age of menopause by 2 years. If, however, smoking stimulates the rate of atresia by only 5%, a similar decrease in age of menopause will occur.

CONCLUSIONS

At the present time it is not known what component of cigarette smoke is producing these adverse reproductive effects. Animal models suggest that at least one component of cigarette smoke, benzo(a)pyrene, is capable of producing effects which are very similar to those seen in women who smoke. Whether benzo(a)pyrene is the only component of cigarette smoke capable of producing reproductive toxicity, or even the most potent, is not known. The data reviewed here provide clear evidence that benzo(a)pyrene, one component of cigarette smoke, is capable of decreasing fertility, altering the frequency of ovulation, and decreasing the reproductive life-span of experimental

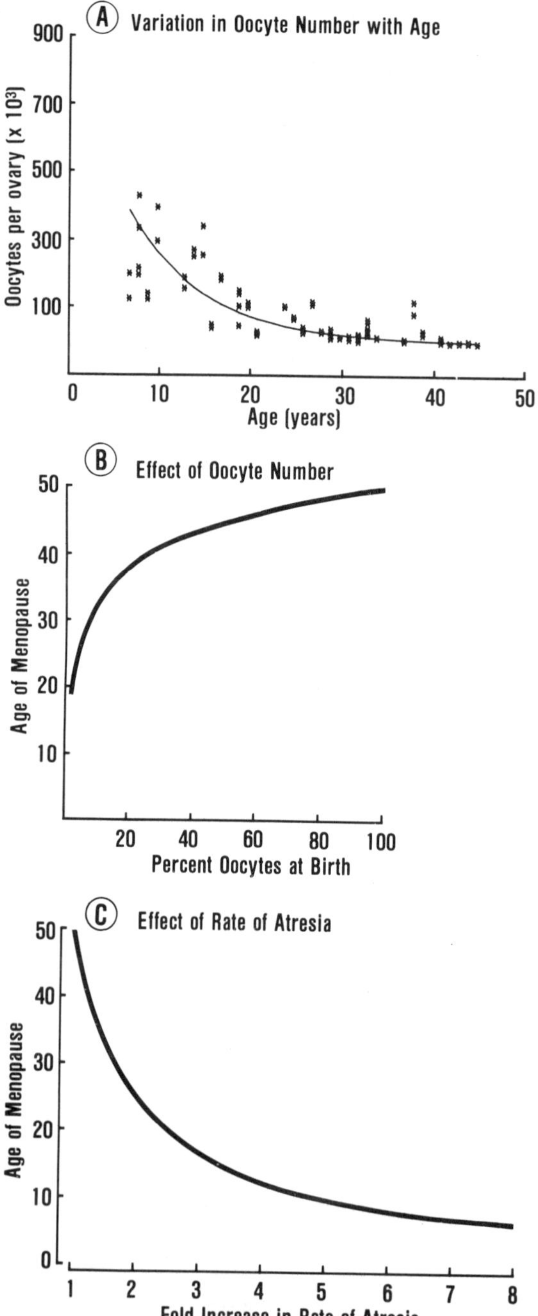

Figure 10-3 Number of oocytes as a function of age.

animals, consistent with the adverse reproductive effects observed among cigarette-smoking women.

REFERENCES

1. Takizawa K, Mattison DR: Female reproduction. *Am J Indust Med* 1983;4:17-30.
2. Dean J: Preimplantation development: biology, genetics and mutagenesis. *Am J Indust Med* 1983;4:31-49.
3. Swartz WJ: Early mammalian embryonic development. *Am J Indust Med* 1983;4:51-61.
4. Hodgen GD: The dominant ovarian follicle. *Fertil Steril* 1982;38:281-300.
5. Mattison DR: The effects of smoking on fertility from gametogenesis to implantation. *Environ Res* 1982;28:410-433.
6. Mattison DR: Clinical manifestations of ovarian toxicity, in Dixon RL (ed): *Reproductive Toxicology*. New York, Raven Press, 1985, pp 109-130.
7. Hammond EC: Smoking in relation to physical complaints. *Arch Environ Health* 1961;3:28-46.
8. Tokuhata GM: Smoking in relation to infertility and fetal loss. *Arch Environ Health* 1968;17:353-359.
9. Baird DD, Wilcox AJ: Cigarette smoking associated with delayed conception. *JAMA* 1985;253:2679-2683.
10. Howe G, Westhoff C, Vessey M, et al: Effects of age, cigarette smoking and other factors on fertility: findings in a large prospective study. *Br Med J* 1985;290:1697-1700.
11. Vessey MP, Wright NH, McPherson K, et al: Fertility after stopping different methods of contraception. *Br Med J* 1978;1:265-267.
12. Baron JA: Smoking and estrogen-related disease. *Am J Epidemiol* 1984;119:9-22.
13. Adena MA, Gallagher HG: Cigarette smoking and the age of menopause. *Ann Hum Biol* 1982;9:121-130.
14. Jick H, Parker J, Morrison AS: Relation between smoking and age of natural menopause. *Lancet* 1977;1:1354-1355.
15. Mattison DR, White NB, Nightingale MS: The effect of benzo(a)pyrene on fertility, primordial number and ovarian response to pregnant mares serum gonadotropin. *Pediatr Pharmacol* 1980;1:143-151.
16. Swartz WJ, Mattison DR: Benzo(a)pyrene inhibits ovulation in C57BL/6N mice. *Anat Rec* 1985;212:268-276.
17. Lu AYH, West SB: Multiplicity of mammalian microsomal cytochromes P-450. *Pharmacol Rev* 1980;31:277-295.
18. Gram TE (ed): *Extrahepatic Metabolism of Drugs and Other Foreign Compounds*. New York and London, SP Medical and Scientific Books, 1980.
19. Mattison DR, Nightingale MS, Shiromizu K: Effects of toxic substances on female reproduction. *Environ Health Perspect* 1983;48:43-52.
20. MacMahon B, Trichopoulus D, Cole P, et al: Cigarette smoking and urinary estrogens. *N Engl J Med*1982;307:1062-1065.
21. Mittler JC, Pogach L, Ertel NH: Effects of chronic smoking on metabolism in dogs. *J Steroid Biochem* 1982;18:759-763.

22. Jasko WJ: Role of tobacco smoking in pharmacokinetics. *J Pharmacokinet Biopharm* 1978;6:7-35.
23. Crawford FE, Back DJ, Orme MLE, et al: Oral contraceptive steroid plasma concentrations in smokers and non-smokers. *Br Med J* 1981;282:1829-1830.
24. Block E: Quantitative morphological investigations of the follicular system in women. Variations at different ages. *Acta Anat* 1952;14:108-123.

11 *Does Smoking Affect Sperm?*

Michael J. Rosenberg

Cigarette smoke contains numerous compounds that induce changes in cellular genetic material and cause cancer in animal bioassays.[1,2] These substances, which are inhaled through active or passive smoking and carried by blood to every tissue in the body, are associated with DNA damage and chromosomal abnormalities in tissues with rapid cellular turnover.[3,4] Blood is richly supplied to the testes by the pampiniform plexus of vessels, where it bathes the cells that produce sperm. Since this tissue is one of the most rapidly growing in the body, it may be particularly susceptible to genetic or other insult.

Smoking is associated with a growing list of medical problems, with attention most recently focused on reproduction. Women who smoke have greater difficulty becoming pregnant than do nonsmokers,[5] but the influence of paternal smoking has been examined in only two studies.[5,6] Although no effect of paternal smoking was found, neither study was designed to investigate this question, and both were limited by the amount of information collected on the men. In the absence of suitable epidemiologic studies, the question of whether paternal smoking impairs the ability to impregnate might be examined by investigating the postulated mechanisms.

A considerable body of literature on male reproductive function suggests that any such impairment would involve two links: first, that smoking adversely affects sperm, and second, that impaired sperm are associated with decreased probability of conception. The existence of the second link is suggested by mounting evidence demonstrating that sperm is an indicator of reproductive impairment.[7] Although papers also exist to suggest a lack of association, the weight of evidence favors the existence of such a relationship. The first link, whether smoking affects sperm quality, is the subject of this review.

BACKGROUND AND METHODS

Sperm are evaluated according to the number of cells per cubic millimeter (density, concentration, or count), the percentage of cells that move (motility), and the percentage that are shaped normally (morphology).[7] Density is measured either by a cell counter (such as the Coulter counter) or manually with a grid-scored microscope slide. The process is easy to perform and is associated with low variability between observers and between laboratories. Motility is generally assessed by estimating the proportion of motile sperm at some fixed period after specimen collection. This tends to be a more subjective measure and is reflected by moderate variability among observers and among laboratories. Sperm morphology, or the percentage of sperm that are normally shaped, is evaluated by classifying the abnormalities according to several schemes. Morphology, which may reflect DNA "packaging," may be the best single indicator of reproductive function. It has low variability from one observer to another but, because of lack of standardization in classifying abnormalities, tends to vary widely among laboratories. Since the methods for these evaluations vary among laboratories, comparing sperm morphology studies is difficult.

In summarizing studies, relative risk is calculated by comparing the proportion of samples with abnormal results in the smokers' group, as defined by each author, relative to the proportion abnormal in nonsmokers. Thus, a relative risk greater than 1.0 means a higher proportion of abnormal results among the smokers group. Variability is indicated by 90% confidence intervals. A confidence interval that does not include 1.0 corresponds with an observed level of statistical significance of $P \leq .10$. In some cases, recalculation from published figures was necessary.

RESULTS

The results of 14 evaluations of the influence of smoking on sperm density, motility, and morphology are summarized in 12 papers (Table 11-1).[8-19] Subjects in these evaluations are most commonly drawn from infertility clinics (in seven evaluations); four studies are based on presumably normal men (healthy volunteers, vasectomy candidates, or sperm donors). Evaluations of men from vasectomy candidates are included in one study, and infertility clinic patients are included in another.[16] In one study, nonsmokers of proven fertility are compared with smokers of unproven fertility.[8] All are cross-sectional designs in which the sperm of smokers and nonsmokers were examined at a single point in time. Sample sizes range from 25 smokers and 20 nonsmokers to 1377 smokers and 580 nonsmokers.

Table 11-1
Results of Evaluations of Influence of Smoking on Sperm Density, Motility, and Morphology

				Sperm Density (10^6/mL)			Motility (%)			Morphology (% normal)		
Authors	Study Group	No. of Subjects	Sample Source	Mean	Relative Risk*	*P*-value†	Mean	Relative Risk*	*P*-value†	Mean	Relative Risk*	*P* – value†
Viczian (1969)[8]	Smokers	120	Volunteers	61			53			73		
	Nonsmokers	50	Volunteers of proven fertility	74			69			81		
Schirrwen and Gey (1969)[9]	Smokers	1,377			1.2			1.0				
	Nonsmokers	580										
Campbell and Harrison (1979)[10]	Smokers	134	Infertility clinic		1.6 (1.2-2.1)			1.3 (1.0-1.9)				
	Nonsmokers	119										
Vogel et al (1979)[11]	Smokers	17	Not Specified		2.1 (1.4-3.3)		65.4		0.2			NS
	Nonsmokers	39					75.0					
Evans et al (1981)[12]	Smokers	43	Infertility clinic						>0.5	52.9	1.4 (1.1-1.7)	
	Nonsmokers	43								57.7		
Godfrey (1981)[13]	Smokers	75	Infertility clinic			>.05			>0.5	61.6		.05
	Nonsmokers	74								65.4		
Rodriguez-Rigau et al (1982)[14]	Smokers	58	Infertility clinic; excludes men with varicocele	55.5	0.9 (0.6-1.5)		58.5		>.05	44.8		<.05
	Nonsmokers	101		52.4			58.4			44.7		

	Smokers	38	Infertility clinic: men with varicocele only	52.3	0.9 (0.6-1.4)	60.3	>.05	44.0	>.05
	Nonsmokers	59		53.2		52.6		42.1	
Shaaraway and Mahmcnd (1982)[15]	Smokers	25	Health volunteers of unproven fertility	74.8	>0.5	52.0	<.0005	52.0	<.0005
	Nonsmokers	20		80.8		78.0		75.0	
Spira (1981)[16]	Smokers	122	Vasectomy candidates	83.8	<.01	52.4	<.05	48.2	NS
	Nonsmokers	173		112.1		56.2		51.2	
	Smokers	292	Infertility clinic	67.0	NS	48.8	NS	40.2	<.02
	Nonsmokers	228		78.3		50.3		44.1	
Handelsman et al (1984)[17]	Smokers	71	Healthy sperm donors	64.1	NS	67.0	.001	73.4	NS
	Nonsmokers	23		95.5		72.0		74.8	
Kulikauskas et al (1985)[18]	Smokers	103	Infertility clinic and premarital exam	55.5	<.001	49.3	<.001	73.0	.09
	Nonsmokers	135		27.3		63.2		74.3	
Vogt et al (1986)[19]	Smokers	150	Healthy volunteers	59.0	.07	73.0	NS	68.8	
	Nonsmokers	52		72.9		74.0		68.0	

From Stillman RJ, Rosenberg MJ, Sachs BP: Smoking and reproduction. *Fertil Steril* 1986;46:545-566. Reproduced wi h permission of the publisher, The American Fertility Society.[21]

* Risk of abnormal result in smokers as compared to nonsmokers.

† Difference between means.

NS = Nonsignificant

Sperm density is reduced in smokers in 11 of the 12 evaluations in which means were reported; density was approximately equal for smokers and nonsmokers in the other study. Density averaged 22% lower in smokers than in nonsmokers, with the greatest reduction being 57%. The risk of low sperm density was slightly more than twice as high for smokers as for nonsmokers in one study[11] and about one and one-half times higher in two other studies;[9,10] in each case, the risks were significant. Relative risks of 0.9, neither of which was significant, were reported in two components of one study.[14] In one study, in which a slightly reduced mean density among smokers was found, a smaller proportion of smokers than nonsmokers had fewer than 20 million sperm/mL.[14] Thus, smokers have a lower mean density than nonsmokers but have a risk of low density of 0.9 compared with nonsmokers.

Additional information on how smoking affects sperm density comes from examining dose response and cessation. Of two studies that include dose response information, a strong inverse relationship between density and level of smoking (0, <20, and ≥ 20 cigarettes per day associated with 55.5, 54.4, and 51.8 x 10^6/mL, respectively) was found in one;[14] an equivocal relationship was found in the other.[8] In another investigation, dramatic increases in sperm density were noted in three men who stopped smoking[11]: while they were smoking, their mean density was 5.2 x 10^6/mL; 6 months after they stopped, their mean density was 47.3 x 10^6/mL. In an additional study, lower density was found among smokers than nonsmokers and intermediate levels were found among men who had quit smoking at least a year before the evaluation.[19]

Of 12 studies in which sperm motility was evaluated, a lower proportion of motile sperm in smokers than in nonsmokers was found in eight, a higher proportion in two, and approximately equal proportions in two. In an additional study, only a nonsignificant difference was reported between the two groups. In the studies that reflect impairment among smokers, the mean percentage of motile sperm was 20% lower among smokers; the studies reflecting better motility among smokers averaged an 11% increase. Two studies reflect slightly increased relative risk of abnormally low motility, one not significant and the other of borderline significance. Increasing levels of smoking were associated with decreased motility in one study[8] and not associated in another.[14] Among three men who stopped smoking, the average number of sperm with "very good" motility improved from 27% to 45%.[9] The motility of former smokers did not differ from that of smokers or nonsmokers in another study.[19]

The proportion of sperm with normal morphology was evaluated in 12 studies. A lower proportion of normally shaped sperm in smokers than in nonsmokers was reported in seven studies, an increase was found in one, and approximately equal proportions were found in four. The magnitude of decrease averaged 17%; the single study in which an increase was found was 5% higher. In the only study in which relative risk was included, smokers were found to be 1.4 times more likely to have a low proportion of normal sperm as nonsmokers. Of the four evaluations of dose response relationships, fewer normally shaped cells were found to be associated with increasing use of cigarettes in two,[8,13] and no association was found in the other two.[12,14]

DISCUSSION

These studies reflect a clear consensus that cigarette smoke impairs sperm concentration, motility, and morphology. Although the decreases are not great, they nonetheless suggest impairments that are sufficient to be clinically apparent. The strength and consistency of impairments (22% for density, 20% for motility, and 17% for morphology for the studies in which an impairment was demonstrated) and the variety of methods used in different studies suggest that chance is an unlikely explanation for these findings. On the other hand, authors of the few studies that inconsistently reflect minimal improvements in the quality of smokers' sperm (2% for density, 11% for motility, and 4% for morphology) argue that these findings are more likely attributable to chance.

The strength and consistency of impairment are not as clearly evident from the conclusions of each paper's authors as from this examination of the collective literature. Part of the divergence is attributable to reliance on tests of significance as indicators of whether the results are meaningful, but it also underscores the diversity of methodologic approaches to the question of whether smoking affects sperm. The strengths and weaknesses of an individual study not only affects its credibility but also makes distinction between an acceptable and unacceptable study difficult. Although the findings described herein reflect this author's review and, in some cases, reanalysis, these summaries are of necessity brief. Because the issues of selection, conduct, and evaluation are central to a study's validity, the following discussion considers these points.

Selection

Nearly all studies involve populations appropriate to the question of whether smoking affects sperm, but additional details would provide reassurance that subjects were selected appropriately. Most studies involve subjects from infertility clinics, so results may not be generalizable to other groups; one author studied groups of smokers and nonsmokers from men seeking attention for infertility and another group from men prior to vasectomy, allowing comparison among all four groups. Since approximately a third of infertility can be attributed to the male partner and a third to neither partner, the studies' external validity would be strengthened by selecting only men whose partners' problems explained the infertility, so that the men are presumably normal. This reassurance was provided in some studies.

One study compared smokers of unknown fertility with nonsmokers of proven fertility.[8] Since men with impaired fertility were excluded from the latter group, this study is strongly biased toward finding impaired sperm in smokers. Although the study found impairments of 18% in density, 23% in motility, and 10% in morphology in the sperm of smokers, these findings were not the most marked of studies reviewed.

In most studies, men were excluded if they had histories or conditions that may have affected their sperm. These include recent febrile illness, certain medications, excessive alcohol use, and exposure to radiation. Men with varicoceles were generally excluded, but separate evaluations of men with and without varicoceles were included in one study. (Values for all parameters were found to be similar to those of men without varicoceles.) This restriction is one way to assure that both groups being compared are free from one form of bias.

Sample size

The number of subjects is a key determinant of a study's ability to detect any difference between the sperm of smokers and nonsmokers. Since significance tests reflect both the magnitude of the difference between samples as well as the number of subjects, a lack of significance can result from studying a small number of subjects, even though they differ markedly in sperm characteristics. When studies lack adequate numbers of subjects, nonsignificant *P*-values may be misinterpreted as unimportant differences.[20] The largest study of sperm density, for example, involves 1377 smokers and 580 nonsmokers[9]; the smallest has 25 smokers and 20 nonsmokers.[15] The large study has a 68% chance of detecting a difference in mean density of 10×10^6/mL, but the smaller study has only a 7% chance (assuming a two-sided alpha of 0.05). For a 5% difference in the morphology of the sperm of smokers and nonsmokers, the largest study (292 smokers, 228 nonsmokers[16]) has a 98% chance of detection; the smaller study has a 20% chance.

Statistical Treatment

In most studies, the *T*-test was used to test for significance between means in all three parameters evaluated. However, this test assumes that values are normally distributed. Most authors who applied the *T*-test did not indicate whether this assumption of normality was appropriate. If data are not normally distributed, as is generally the case for density, then the data can be transformed to normality, or a nonparametric test (such as the Mann-Whitney test) can be used.

Evaluation and treatment of potential confounders

Factors that affect sperm (such as those listed under "Selection") and are more common in one group being compared are termed confounders. They may distort the comparison between smokers and nonsmokers, resulting in misleading conclusions. In none of the studies was evaluation included of whether such factors that were not a basis for exclusion may have distorted the comparison. Although the list of factors potentially influencing one or more sperm parameters is long and subject to interpretation, in nearly all studies men were included who had at least one factor that was the basis for exclusion in another. Standard techniques to adjust for such unequal distribution include stratification and multivariate analysis, such as analysis of covariance. In these studies, no such adjustments were performed, nor were there assurances that they were unnecessary. For example, a factor that strongly influences sperm concentration, the abstinence period prior to specimen collection, is not mentioned in any of these papers.

Clinical significance

Although smoking impairs the production of normal sperm, assessment of the clinical impact of smoking awaits studies specifically designed to evaluate the issue. The changes reflected by this literature are not great, but they do suggest that men who smoke have fewer sperm that move less efficiently and have a higher proportion of abnormally shaped sperm than do nonsmoking men. The likely impact of these impairments is to decrease the probability of conception. This effect may be subtle and of greatest importance in the event of marginal ability to conceive, analogous to the decreased probability of conception found in women who smoke. This effect must, however, remain conjecture until studies specifically designed to evaluate the effect of paternal smoking on the ability to conceive are conducted.

REFERENCES

1. US Dept of Health and Human Services: *The Health Consequences of Smoking.* A Report of the Surgeon General. Government Printing Office, 1982.
2. Hoffmann D, Hecht SS: Nicotine-derived N-nitrosamines and tobacco-related cancer: Current status and future directions. *Cancer Res* 1985;45:935-944.
3. Hopkin JM, Evans HJ: Cigarette smoke-induced DNA damage and lung cancer risks. *Nature* 1980;283:388-390.

4. Everson RB, Randerath E, Santella RM, et al: Detection of smoking-related covalent DNA adducts in human placenta. *Science* 1986;231:54-57.
5. Baird DD, Wilcox AJ: Cigarette smoking associated with delayed conception. *JAMA* 1985;353:2979-2983..
6. Tokuhata GK: Smoking in relation to infertility and fetal loss. *Arch Environ Health* 1968;17:353-359.
7. Wyrobek AJ, Gordon LA, Burkhart JC, et al: Evaluation of sperm as indicators of chemically induced alterations of spermatogenic function: A report of the US Environmental Protection gene-tox program. *Mutat Res* 1983;115:73-148.
8. Viczian M: Ergebnisse von Spermauntersuchungen bei Zigarettenraunchern. *Z Haut Geschlkr* 1969;44:183-187.
9. Schirren C, Gey G: Der Einfluss des Rauchens and die Fortpflanzungsfähigkeit bei Mann and Frau. *Z Haut Geschlkr* 1969;44:175-182.
10. Campbell JM, Harrison KL: Smoking and infertility. *Med J Austr* 1979;1:342-343.
11. Vogel W, Broverman DM, Klaiber EL: Gonadal, behavioral, and electroencephalographic correlates of smoking, in Remond A, Izard C (eds): *Electrophysiological Effects of Nicotine.* Amsterdam, Elsevier Biomedical Press, 1979, pp 201-215.
12. Evans HJ, Fletcher J, Torrance M: Sperm abnormalities and cigarette smoking. *Lancet* 1981;1:627-629.
13. Godfrey B: Sperm morphology in smokers. *Lancet* 1981;1:948.
14. Rodriguez-Rigau LJ, Smith KD, Steinberger E: Cigarette smoking and semen quality. *Fertil Steril* 1982;38:115-116.
15. Shaaraway M, Mahmoud, KZ: Endocrine profile and semen characteristics in male smokers. *Fertil Steril* 1982;38:255-257.
16. Spira A: Consummation de tabac et caractéristique du sperme, in Jouannet P, Spira A (eds): *Human Fertility Factors with Emphasis on the Male.* Paris, Institut National de la Santé et de la Recherche Medicale, 1981, pp 363-372.
17. Handelsman DJ, Conway AJ, Boylan LM, et al: Testicular function in potential sperm donors: normal ranges and the effects of smoking and varicocoele. *Int J Androl* 1984;7:369-382.
18. Kulikauskas V, Blaustein D, Ablin RJ: Cigarette smoking and its possible effects on sperm. *Fertil Steril* 1985;44:526-528.
19. Vogt HJ, Heller WD, Borelli S: Sperm quality of healthy smokers, ex-smokers, and never-smokers. *Fertil Steril* 1986;45:106-110.
20. Rothman KJ: A show of confidence. *N Engl J Med* 1978;299:1362-1363.
21. Stillman RJ, Sachs BP, Rosenberg MJ : Smoking and reproduction. *Fertil Steril* 1986;46:545-566.

12 *Smoking and Fecundity*

Alfred Spira, Jacque de Mouzan, Samuel Schwartz

Fecundity, or the ability to achieve pregnancy, is defined as the probability of conception for a given couple during a given menstrual cycle[1] (fertility denotes having produced a child). This probability can, in turn, be expressed as the product of three independent probabilities[2]:

$$P = P_o \times P_f \times P_{ve}$$

where P_o = probability of ovum production
P_f = probability of fertilization of this ovum by spermatozoa
P_{ve} = probability that the egg is viable.

The effect of smoking on fecundity can be directly studied with cohort or case-control studies. The literature, however, provides important clues about the effects of smoking on each of the three components of fecundity. Review reveals three well-documented considerations:

1. Elements of cigarette smoke may adversely affect the regulatory mechanisms of the hypothalamic-pituitary-ovarian axis, which may explain the increased frequency of menstrual abnormalities in women who smoke.[3]
2. Spermatogenesis and other aspects of testicular function may be altered by smoking.[4] The ability of the spermatozoa to reach the ovum depends on both motility and tubal patency.
3. Maternal cigarette smoking significantly increases the rate of spontaneous abortions, mainly of fetuses with normal karyotypes.[5]

These well-established results lead to the logical conclusion that smoking women, and perhaps smoking men, might have reduced fecundity. The review of the literature, however, indicates that the actual situation is more complicated.

LITERATURE ON SMOKING, FECUNDITY, AND FERTILTY

Of ten published[6-15] and one unpublished studies (Table 12-1), only seven show an increased risk of infertility or low fecundity in smokers. These studies reported relative risks (RRs), or odds ratios, between 1.3 and 1.6, except in one study[12] where it is 3.3. The corresponding attributable risk, however, is greater, with 23% and 37%, respectively, of fecundity impairment attributable to smoking. Fecundity among smokers thus appears to be decreased, but the relationship is weak. This discordance may be due to different methods or may reflect a real but slight increased risk in smokers.

Tokuhata[6] studied women who had died of cancer of the reproductive system or the breast and whose family members provided information about smoking exposure. This study showed increased risk of infertility among smokers. The relationship between smoking and certain cancers of the reproductive system is now well established, making this sample's validity rather suspicious. No information is provided about any dose-response relationship between smoking and low fecundity.

Friedman[7] studied a cohort of women entering a program of artificial insemination with semen donors and found no effect of smoking on fecundity. However, no details of methodology used to study the issue are provided, and the sample is very small and may not be representative of a larger population (the women were very concerned by the couple's failure to conceive, which was due to the husband's infertility).

Mai et al[8] conducted a psychiatric study of 50 couples who had been referred to an infertility clinic and 50 women assumed to be fertile. The results suggest an association of smoking with infertility: the infertile women had significantly more variability in cigarettes smoked per day. For infertile women the standard deviation was 6.27; for the fertile women it was 4.85 ($P < .05$). Both this difference and the higher average daily consumption by the infertile group (7.8 compared with 7.0 cigarettes per day) are due to heavy smoking by a few of the infertile wives, raising the possibility that the results are skewed by a small number of heavy smokers.

Linn et al[9] conducted a retrospective study of 3214 women having planned pregnancies and singleton deliveries who had no history of infertility treatment and who conceived more than 2 weeks after cessation of contraception. In this study, the interval between cessation of contraception and conception was calculated by subtracting the length of gestation from the time since last use of contraception. Although this method is rather crude, it does not introduce any bias in the comparison between smokers and nonsmokers. The risk of infertility among smokers compared with nonsmokers was 1.0 (95% confidence interval [CI] = 0.9-1.2).

Olsen et al[10] studied 1069 women treated for infertility and a control group of 4305 women who had delivered healthy children at the same hospital

Table 12-1
Smoking and Fecundity

Author(s)	Study Design.	Sample Size	Adjusted RR (if applicable) (95% CI)	Potential Confounders controlled
Tokuhata (1968)[6]	Retrospective cohort	2016	1.5	Cause of death, age education, occupation, tobacco use by husband
Friedman (1972)[7]	Cohort	227	1.0	None
Mai et al (1977)[8]	Case-control	100	>1.0	None
Linn et al (1982)[9]	Retrospective cohort	32	1.0 (0.9-1.2)	Contraception, age, parity, body mass, education, pelvic inflammatory disease
Olsen et al (1982)[10]	Case-control	4655	1.6 (1.1-2.2)	Alcohol, contraception, age, residence, education, parity
Harlap (1984)[11]	Retrospective cohort	5880	1.0	None
Daling (1985)[12]	Case-control	1181	3.3 (1.9-5.6)	Race, residence, age (matched)
Cramer (1985)[13]	Case-control	4411* 5515†	1.6 (1.3-2.0) 1.1 (1.0-1.2)	Age, race, payment status
Baird (1984)[14]	Retrospective cohort	678	1.4 (1.1-1.7)	Age, parity, infertility, intercourse freq., oral contraception, recent pregnancy, alcohol, body mass
Howe (1985)[15]	Retrospective cohort	4104	1.3 (1.1-1.4)	Contraception, age
de Mouzon (unpublished data, 1985)	Retrospective cohort	1576	1.1 (0.8-1.7)	Contraception, parity, occupation, reference year

*Tubal disease: †Nontubal disease.

during the same period. The relation between smoking and infertility is significant for comparison of control subjects with the group of infertile women whose medical histories were potentially related to smoking or drinking or for whom no medical reason could be found to account for their infertility. Odds ratios were 1.6 (1.1-2.2) for impaired fecundity among women who had never been pregnant and 2.1 (1.3-3.6) for impaired fecundity after at least one pregnancy. The relation is also significant for the comparison of fertile couples who had a delay in conception of more than 1 year with the rest of the fertile group (odds ratio 1.8 (1.3-2.5) for impaired fecundity among women never pregnant and 1.3 (1.0-1.8) for women who had been pregnant previously.

In another part of the analysis, couples were used as controls whose infertility was diagnosed as "unlikely to have been directly caused by smoking or drinking: displaced testis, varicocele, mumps as an adult (male), blocked fallopian tubes, etc..." In this part of the study, the odds ratios for smoking were 0.8 (0.5, 1.1) for primary subfecundity and 1.0 (0.5, 1.8) for secondary subfecundity. Moreover, significantly more women with blocked fallopian tubes were smokers ($P < .05$) than were women with other medical histories "probably not tobacco related." This is the first report of a possible relationship between smoking and tubal disease; the results show clearly that the most important part of the relationship between smoking and infertility disappears when the data are adjusted for tubal disease.

Harlap and Baras[11] studied retrospectively delay in conception among 1403 women who stopped oral contraceptives in order to conceive and 4477 control subjects who stopped using other contraceptives. They note that smoking had no effect on fertility and found no obvious interaction of the pill with smoking.

Daling et al[12] studied primary tubal infertility in relation to the use of an intrauterine device. Of the 549 women with primary infertility who were interviewed, smoking status was available only for the 172 who had a diagnosis of tubal infertility. Of these, 37.7% were smokers, but only 15.7% of the matched controls smoked (RR = 3.3 (1.9-5.6)). By far, this represents the strongest reported effect of smoking on reducing fertility. This is also the only study limited to cases with diagnosed tubal disease.

The design of the study by Cramer et al[13] is quite similar to that of Daling et al,[12] but data about smoking status are available separately for all cases and for women with tubal disease. When women consulting physicians for infertility due to tubal occlusion are considered, the odds ratio for smokers compared with nonsmokers is 1.6 (1.3-2.0) compared with controls matched for age, race, and payment status in the same hospitals. When women consulting for infertility unrelated to tubal disease are considered, the odds ratio for smoking is only 1.1 (1.0-1.2). Although the studies were not designed to examine the relationship between smoking and fecundity, these two papers stress the link between smoking and tubal disease.

In a retrospective study, Baird and Wilcox[14] collected data from 678 pregnant women on their smoking history and number of unprotected cycles until conception. After the data were adjusted for potential confounding variables, the fertility of smokers was estimated to be 72% of that of nonsmokers (RR = 1.4 (1.1-1.7)). Although this study may overestimate the effects of smoking,[16] the fertility of light smokers (<20 cigarettes per day) was found to be 75% of that of nonsmokers. In addition, the fertility of heavy smokers (>20 cigarettes per day) was observed to be 57% of that of nonsmokers, but this trend did not achieve statistical significance. The authors also indicate that they could find no association between history of pelvic infection and fertility.

Howe et al[15] report data from the prospective Oxford Family Planning Association study, which show decreased fertility for cigarette smokers after age, last method of contraception, and time since stopping contraception are taken into account. However, this consistent, highly significant trend of decreasing fertility with increasing number of cigarettes smoked per day occurs only in women smoking 16 to 20 cigarettes per day (relative fertility rate = 0.79) or more than 20 cigarettes per day (relative fertility rate = 0.78). For lighter smokers, the decrease in fertility rate is not significant. The authors stress that in the Oxford Family Planning Association study, cigarette smoking was related to an increased incidence of pelvic inflammatory disease. However, this disease was rare among the study participants, and the association does not explain the decreased relative fertility rates observed in heavy smokers.

Finally, in a prospective cohort study undertaken in France of 1576 couples, the authors, using a Cox proportional hazards regression model, could show no decrease in fecundity in smokers after the data were adjusted for confounders (deMouzon J, personal communication, June 1985).

OVERVIEW AND QUESTIONS

1. The increased relative risk associated with smoking by women, although significant and very well documented in some studies, is weak in these (under 1.6 in all but one study).

2. The relationship does not seem to be dose related, although this problem was examined in only two studies[14,15] and spuriously found to be significant in one of them.[15]

3. Howe et al[15] stress that "the dose-response relationship between smoking and the relative fertility rates certainly suggests a causal relation." This conclusion is supported when all data from the literature are analyzed according to the general criteria for establishing causation[16]:

a. Strength of Association: The association is weak.

b. Dose-response effect: There is no proof.

c. Lack of temporal ambiguity: Usually people begin to smoke early in life, at least before they try to conceive. However, as pointed out by Mai et al,[8] infertile wives exhibit significantly more hysterical and aggressive personality disorders, which may be accompanied by increased smoking.

d. Consistency of the findings: Only seven of 11 published studies demonstrate a clear relationship. Not only is a causal hypothesis not supported, but the studies also stress the importance of two factors related to both smoking and infecundity that were not considered in any of the studies, namely sexual behavior and pelvic inflammatory disease (PID).

e. Biological plausibility of the hypothesis and coherence of the evidence: The hypothesis is fairly plausible. Moreover, the prevalence of regular cigarette smoking among women has been increasing since 1976,[17] and at the same time the infertility incidence has increased.[18] But this increase in incidence is generally reported to be related to the growing incidence of PID, which may be related to smoking.

f. The specificity of the association: Smoking is not associated only with infertility, and infertility is related to many other factors independent of smoking.

Thus only two of the six general criteria used to assess causal interpretation are met for smoking and infertility.

5. The sexual behavior of smokers differs from that of nonsmokers. Malcom and Shephard[19] studied the reported sexual behavior of adolescents in relation to smoking habits and found that female smokers tend to date more often than nonsmokers (85% *v* 54%) and that male smokers have more sexual partners (in 62% of cases *v* 3%) and have intercourse more often than nonsmokers. One of the major risk factors for sexually transmitted disease (STD) is high number of sexual partners. Pelvic inflammatory disease is a frequent complication of STD, and infertility results from about 15% of cases of PID.[20] The reported high incidence of PID[15] and tubal diseases[10,12] in smokers supports this hypothesis. Another argument in its favor is that the highest relative risk of infertility among smokers was reported in the study of Daling et al,[12] in which only tubal diseases are studied, and that in the study of Cramer et al[13] the odds ratio is significantly higher than in the study of Daling et al. There is usually a very close relationship between husband's and wife's smoking (deMouzon J, personal communication, June 1985), and male smokers are at greater risk of urethritis than are nonsmokers.[21,22]

CONCLUSIONS

Existing data permit conclusions that:

1. A relationship exists between smoking and spontaneous abortions and possibly gamete production, but the effect of smoking on fecundity is not clear.

2. Smokers seem to be at greater risk than nonsmokers for infections of the reproductive tract. However, it is unclear whether this is the result of different lifestyles, changes in immune response, or both.[23] The reported relation between smoking and reduced fecundity may be only artifactual and explained by confounders which have not been taken into account. In the only study in which the data were adjusted for behavioral factors (deMuzon J, personal communication, June 1985), no effect of smoking could be shown.

REFERENCES

1. Gini C: Proceedings of the Mathematics Congress. Toronto, 1924; p 889.
2. Schwartz D, MacDonald P, Heuchel V: Fecundability, coital frequency and the viability of ova. *Popul Stud* 1980;34:397-400.
3. Mattison DR: The effects of smoking on fertility from gametogenesis to implantation. *Environ Res* 1982;28:410-433.
4. Rosenberg MJ: Does smoking affect sperm? in Rosenberg MJ (ed): *Smoking and Reproductive Health.* Littleton, Mass, PSG Publishing Co, 1987.
5. Hasselmeyer EG, Meyer MB, Longo LD, et al: Pregnancy and infant health, in *The Health Consequences of Smoking for Women. A Report of the Surgeon General.* US Dept of Health and Human Services, Government Printing Office, 1983, pp 189-249.
6. Tokuhata G: Smoking in relation to infertility and fetal loss. *Arch Environ Health* 1968;17:353-359.
7. Friedman S: Artificial donor insemination with frozen human semen. *Fertil Steril* 1977;28:1230-1233.
8. Mai FM, Munday RN, Rump EE: Psychiatric interview comparisons between infertile and fertile couples. *Psychosom Med* 1972;34:431-440.
9. Linn S, Schoenbaum SC, Monson RR, et al: Delay in conception for former "pill" users. *JAMA* 1982;247:629-632.
10. Olsen J, Rachootin P, Schiodt AV, et al: Tobacco use, alcohol consumption and infertility. *Int J Epidemiol* 1982;12:179-184.
11. Harlap S, Baras M: Conception-waits in fertile women after stopping oral contraceptives. *Int J Fertil* 1984;29:73-80.
12. Daling JR, Weiss NS, Metch BJ, et al: Primary tubal infertility in relation to the use of an intrauterine device. *N Engl J Med* 1985;312:937-941.
13. Cramer DW, Schiff I, Schoenbaum SC, et al: Tubal infertility and the intrauterine device. *N Engl J Med* 1985;312: 941-947.
14. Baird DD, Wilcox AJ: Cigarette smoking associated with delayed conception. *JAMA* 1984;253:2979-2983.
15. Howe G, Westhoff C, Vessey M, et al: Effects of age, cigarette smoking, and other factors on fertility: findings in a large prospective study. *Br Med J* 1985;290:1697 1700.
16. Kleinbaum DG, Kupper K, Morgenstern H: *Epidemiologic Research—Principles and Quantitative Methods.* London, Lifetime Learning Publications, 1982, pp 32-34.
17. Harris JE: Patterns of cigarette smoking, in *The Health Consequences of Smoking for Women. A Report of the Surgeon General.* US Dept of Health and Human Services, Government Printing Office 1983; pp 17-42.
18. Pratt WF, Mosher WD, Bachrach CA, et al: Understanding U.S. fertility:

Findings from the National Survey of Family Growth, cycle III. *Popul Bull* 1984;5:1-41.
19. Malcom S, Shephard RJ: Personality and sexual behavior of the adolescent smoker. *Am J Drug Alcohol Abuse* 1978;5:87-96.
20. Westrom L: Effects of acute PID in fertility. *Am J Obstet Gynecol* 1975;121:707-713.
21. Boyce A, Schwartz D, David G: Smoking and genitourinary infection. *Br Med J* 1976;2:1013.
22. Martin-Boyce A, David G, Schwartz D: Alcool, tabac et infections génito-urinaires masculines. *Rev Epidemiol Sante Publique* 1977;25:209-216.

13 *Smoking and Ectopic Pregnancy: A Multinational Case-Control Study*

Oona M. Campbell, Ronald H. Gray

A dramatic increase in the incidence of ectopic pregnancy over the past three decades has been noted in developed countries.[1-3] Previous studies of the etiology of ectopic pregnancy focused on physiologic mechanisms such as tubal spasm and menstrual reflux, in addition to the well-established mechanism of pelvic inflammatory disease (PID).[4] To explain the increasing incidence of ectopic pregnancy, recent studies consider factors such as intrauterine device (IUD) use, tubal ligation, induced abortion, and PID, which have also been increasing.[1,3,5,6]

In 1978, the World Health Organization began a multicenter case-control study of ectopic pregnancy. The main objectives were to examine the role of contraceptives in the risk of ectopic pregnancy and to determine what other risk factors, such as PID, are associated with it. In addition, the study was designed to assess whether risk factors for ectopic pregnancy are similar in developed and developing countries.[7,8] One of the most interesting findings was unexpected. A question on women's smoking status (current, former, or never) was included in the questionnaire, although smoking was not hypothesized to be a risk factor. Analysis of the data showed smoking to be a consistent risk factor for ectopic pregnancy.

METHODS

The study was conducted between 1978 and 1980 in 12 centers, eight in developing countries and four in developed countries, with a total of 1108 case-control triplets (927 in developing and 181 in developed countries.) The cases, identified in participating hospitals, were 1108 women with ectopic pregnancies confirmed by histopathologic evidence of fetal tissue or chorionic villi from an extrauterine site. Each case was matched to two controls: (1) a pregnant control identified in an antenatal or preabortion clinic, and (2) a nonpregnant control identified from nonobstetric, nongynecologic admissions. The matching criteria were age, parity, marital status, and date of admission. All cases and controls were interviewed by trained interviewers using a standard questionnaire.

Information on obstetric, gynecologic, and medical history, contraceptive use, and current smoking was obtained. No sexual history was obtained for cultural reasons. Analyses were done separately for pregnant and nonpregnant controls and according to whether the case-control triplets were from developed or developing countries. When the odds ratios were estimated by the Breslow-Day conditional logistic regression for matched pairs,[9] the main risk factors to emerge included IUD use, tubal ligation, history of a prior ectopic pregnancy, and a history of PID or gonorrhea.

RESULTS

The prevalence of current smoking was higher in cases than in either of the two control groups. This was true in all centers, but the difference between cases and controls was greater in developing countries where the prevalence was 16.7% among cases, 6.7% among pregnant controls, and 8.9% among nonpregnant controls. In the developed countries, the percent smoking was 47.0%, 36.5%, and 42.0% respectively. The differences in smoking prevalence seen between cases and controls did not result from controls selectively giving up smoking due to pregnancy or hospitalization, since the ex-smokers were evenly distributed among cases and controls.

The smoking variable was included in a multiple logistic regression to adjust for the other variables (PID, history of ectopic pregnancy, and contraceptive method) known or suspected to affect the risk of ectopic pregnancy (Table 13-1). Smoking is significant in all subgroups except the nonpregnant controls in developed countries. Interaction terms between smoking and other variables were included but were not significant and did not change the risk estimates markedly.

Because the association of smoking with ectopic pregnancy was unexpected, the possibility of bias or confounding was carefully considered. For example, confounding might occur if smoking were associated with a cluster of behaviors, such as increased sexual activity, which in turn is associated with increased PID. Alternatively, if oral contraceptive use were contraindica-

Table 13-1
Adjusted Odds Ratios for Smoking as a Risk Factor for Ectopic Pregnancy

	Pregnant Controls	
	Developing Countries	Developed Countries
Adjusted Smoking Odds Ratio*	4.0	2.2
95% Confidence Limits	(2.7-5.9)	(1.3-3.6)
	Nonpregnant Controls	
Adjusted Smoking Odds Ratio*	2.4	1.1
95% Confidence Limits	(1.6-3.4)	(0.6-1.9)

* Adjusted for history of PID or gonorrhea, prior ectopic pregnancy, use of contraceptives, tubal ligation, and induced abortion.

ted for smokers and these women used the IUD instead, the association with ectopic pregnancy could be due to IUD use rather than smoking. Confounding factors might also explain the differences in risk estimates obtained for developed and developing countries: lower prevalence of smoking in developing countries might, for example, indicate a different pattern of behavior.

Although the multivariate analysis adjusts for PID and other potential confounders, we also stratified to eliminate women with exposures to any of the known risk factors (PID, IUD use, tubal ligation, and prior ectopic pregnancy) (Table 13-2). The elevated risk associated with smoking was still reflected in all groups except the nonpregnant controls in developed countries.

We also examined the distribution of ectopic implantation sites in smoking and nonsmoking cases. The distributions showed a nonsignificant but suggestive increase in proximal implantation sites among smokers (12%) compared with nonsmokers (8%). This trend was consistent in subgroups such as women with no exposures to known risk factors.

Table 13-2
Risk of Ectopic Pregnancy for Smoking Among Women with No Known Risk Factors

	Pregnant Controls	
	Developing Countries	Developed Countries
Smoking Odds Ratio	2.6	1.4
95% Confidence Limits	(1.7-3.9)	(0.7-2.6)
	Nonpregnant Controls	
Smoking Odds Ratio	2.8	0.8
95% Confidence Limits	(1.9-4.2)	(0.7-2.4)

DISCUSSION

The results suggest a causal association between smoking and increased risk of ectopic pregnancy. Several criteria for causality are fulfilled by the data. First, strength of the association is great (odds ratios as high as 4.0 in one developing country subgroup). The relationship is also consistent, with an elevated risk in three of the four groups studied as well as in women with no other exposures to known risk factors.

The data have several limitations, however. The temporal sequence of the relationship must remain speculative, as the women were asked their smoking status at time of the interview and not at the time of conception. A dose-response relationship cannot be determined, since no information was obtained on the amount smoked. The small number of repeat ectopic pregnancies precluded analysis for the effect of smoking on recurrence of the condition. Finally, in the absence of a sexual history, we could not rule out potential confounding by differences in behavior between smokers and nonsmokers.

An important criterion to consider in looking for a direct association is biologic plausibility. We reviewed the literature to see if possible biological mechanisms existed through which smoking could exert a causal effect on ectopic pregnancy. In a review article, Mattison[10] suggests that smoking can affect the reproductive process at any point from gametogenesis to implantation. Specifically, cigarette smoke or nicotine alters the motility of the fallopian tube and may impair implantation of the embryo.

Three papers provide supportive evidence for biologic plausibility. The first two studies used Rubin insufflators to examine tubal motility in women and rhesus monkeys. Women were asked to smoke one cigarette in five minutes, and changes in tubal motility were recorded; the rhesus monkeys were injected with nicotine as well as being induced to smoke.[11,12] Both groups exhibited dramatic changes in tubal motility following exposure to smoke. In a third experiment, in which rats were injected with nicotine, the ova in treated rats divided and entered the uterus more slowly, and the blastocycts implanted much closer to each other and clustered at the distal end of the tube.[13]

Replication of findings is an important consideration for judging plausibility. Although no studies have focused on smoking and ectopic pregnancy, an association between smoking and ectopic pregnancy was an incidental finding in two epidemiologic studies. In a cross-sectional study, Matsunaga and Shiota[14] examined the role of limited physical space in causing localized malformations in the embryo and found an excess of smokers among women with ectopic pregnancy. In a case-control study of ectopic pregnancy by Levin et al,[15], smoking was associated with an increased risk, but the authors considered it to be a confounder and treated the variable as an indicator of lifestyle. One piece of data contradicts the evidence of an association between smoking and ectopic pregnancy: in a prospective study of pregnant women, Swedish researchers found no increase in ectopic gestation among smokers.[16] However, subjects were enrolled into the study late in gestation, after the time most ectopics are diagnosed.

In summary, suggestive evidence from human and animal studies indicates that smoking may increase the risk of extrauterine implantation, possibly by affecting tubal motility. Adjustment for known confounders cannot account for this increased smoking risk in the WHO study. There is a need for further study to examine the dose-response effects of smoking, to establish the smoking status of women at the time of conception, and to adjust for potential confounding by controlling for sexual activity.

REFERENCES

1. Robinson N, Beral V: Risk of ectopic pregnancy. *Lancet* 1979;1:1247-1248.
2. Sivin L: Copper IUD use and ectopic pregnancy rates in the United States. *Contraception* 1979;19:151-173.
3. Westrom L, Bengtsson LPH, Mardh PA: Incidence, trends, and risks of ectopic pregnancy in a population of women. *Br Med J* 1981;282:15-18.
4. Green TH: *Gynecology: Essentials of Clinical Practice*, ed 3. Boston, Little, Brown & Co, 1977.
5. Tatum HJ, Schmidt FK: Contraceptive and sterilization practices and extrauterine pregnancies: a relative perspective. *Fertil Steril* 1977;28:407-421.
6. Panayotou PP, Kaskarelis DB, Miettinen OS: Induced abortion and ectopic pregnancy. *Am J Obstet Gynecol* 1972; 114:507-510.

7. World Health Organization Task Force on Intrauterine Devices for Fertility Regulation: A multi-national case-control study of ectopic pregnancy. *Clin Reprod Fertil* 1985;3:131-143.
8. Gray RH: A case-control study of ectopic pregnancy in developed and developing countries, in Zatuchni GI, Goldsmith A, Sciarra J (eds): *Intrauterine Contraception: Advances and Future Prospects*. PARFR Series on Fertility Regulation. Presented at PARFR Conference, Chicago, May 29-June 1, 1984. Philadelphia, Harper & Row, 1985 pp 354-364.
9. Breslow NE, Day NE: Statistical methods in cancer research. The analysis of case-control studies. *IARC Sci Publ* 1980; No. 32.
10. Mattison DR: The effects of smoking on fertility from gametogenesis to implantation. *Environ Res* 1982;28:410-433.
11. Neri A, Ekerling B: Influence of smoking and adrenaline on the uterotubal insufflation test (Rubin test). *Fertil Steril* 1969;20:818-828.
12. Neri A, Marcus SL: Effect of nicotine on the motility of the oviducts in the rhesus monkey: a preliminary report. *J Reprod Fertil* 1972;31:91-97.
13. Yoshinaga K, Rice C, Krenn J, et al: Effects of nicotine on early pregnancy in the rat. *Biol Reprod* 1979;20:294-305.
14. Matsunaga E, Shiota K: Ectopic pregnancy and myoma uteri: teratogenic effects and maternal characteristics. *Teratology* 1980;21:61-69.
15. Levin AA, Schoenbaum SC, Stubblefield PG, et al: Ectopic pregnancy and prior induced abortion. *Am J Public Health* 1982;72:253-256.
16. Kullander S, Kaellen B: A prospective study of smoking and pregnancy. *Acta Obstet Gynec Scand* 1971;50;83-94.

14 *Smoking and Spontaneous Abortion*

Susan Harlap

Over 40 years ago smoking was seen to be related to spontaneous abortion, both in humans[1,2] and in animals.[3] The association aroused little interest among either gynecologists or public health physicians, and 20 years went by before health researchers paid any attention to the topic. During the 1950s and 1960s, a period of intense activity in perinatal research, large cohort studies of perinatal health were set up in Britain, Canada, and the United States, including the Collaborative Perinatal Project and other studies in California and Hawaii. Concurrently, a number of smaller research groups, often gynecologists, studied more limited groups of patients in selected hospitals. Although interest focused on the effect of smoking on birth weight, fetal growth, obstetric complications, and perinatal mortality, a few researchers attempted to study spontaneous abortions.[4-10]

These early studies of smoking and abortion were seriously flawed according to modern standards of epidemiologic science. Little was then known of the epidemiology of spontaneous abortion, and there was little appreciation of the characteristics of smokers that, independently of smoking, would be likely to affect the chances of an abortion. Consequently, these studies contribute little to our understanding of the subject, other than suggesting that smokers are at increased risk for miscarriage.

Major difficulties in research in this topic include the knowledge that before the laws relating to abortion were changed induced abortion was commonly recorded as spontaneous. Spontaneous abortion does not invariably lead to hospitalization; women aborting may not even seek medical assistance. Women admitted to hospitals may differ from those not admitted in the degree of bleeding or in other health characteristics, some of which could well be related to smoking. Another difficulty arises from the fact that the probability of miscarriage, along with its causes, changes with time.[11,12] Consequently, simpler methods of statistical analysis are not appropriate for studies of this topic. Further problems arise from the need to take into account confounding variables: in most countries smokers and nonsmokers differ in age distribution, social class, education, drinking habits, body fat, use of drugs, and other characteristics, and some of these also alter the frequency of abortions.[12-15] Crude comparisons of abortion rates in smokers and nonsmokers are therefore inappropriate.

In the past decade five research groups, three in the United States and two in Scandinavia, have investigated the relationship between smoking and abortion, taking into account potential confounding variables. Kullander and Kallen[16] studied 6363 pregnancies prospectively, defining spontaneous abortion as termination of a pregnancy before the eighth month of gestation. The crude relative risk of spontaneous abortion in their study group was 1.4. These researchers noted an association between smoking and unwanted pregnancy, women with unwanted pregnancies being more often smokers and smoking more heavily. Recalculating the published data shows relative risks of 1.2 and 1.6 for abortion in smokers with wanted and unwanted pregnancies, respectively. The authors suggested that the larger excess risk in the unwanted pregnancies was explained by induced abortions incorrectly reported as spontaneous. Induced abortions were also associated with smoking. (When this study was done induced abortion was restricted in Sweden.)

In New York, Kline et al[17] conducted a carefully controlled retrospective study comparing women having spontaneous abortions with women delivering after 28 weeks of gestation. They found a statistically significant association between smoking and miscarriage, with an odds ratio of 1.8. This association did not vary with age or previous obstetric events.

Himmelberger et al[18] used a mailed questionnaire to conduct a retrospective study of American women health workers. They also found a statistically significant excess of smoking in women reporting spontaneous abortions, even after the data were adjusted for age, exposure to trace anesthetic gases, pregnancy history, and mailing response. The association did not vary with age, exposure to anesthetic gases, or pregnancy history.

In a somewhat similar survey in Finland, Hemminki et al[19] found relative risks of 1.2 and 1.7 in light and heavy smokers respectively (1-10 and >10 cigarettes/day) in surgical nurses, after the data were adjusted for age, parity, and alcohol and coffee use. In workers who sterilize instruments the adjusted relative risks were 0.3 and 1.3 for light and heavy smokers, respectively. These differences were not statistically significant, but the study involved only small numbers of pregnancies.

In a large cohort study in California, Harlap and Shiono[20] investigated the effects of alcohol on spontaneous abortion and pointed out that, since alcohol use and smoking tend to be strongly correlated, alcohol must be controlled for in studies dealing with the effects of smoking on pregnancy outcome. After taking into account other confounding variables, the researchers concluded that the relative risk of smoking 1.5 packs or more daily was less than that associated with drinking, being 1.1 in nondrinkers, 1.9 in light drinkers, and 1.0 in heavy drinkers.

The California study also investigated the effects of smoking at different periods of gestation and found no obvious difference between the first and the second trimester. This finding was unexpected, since the causes of miscarriage vary with gestational age. Early abortions are most often associated with chromosomal abnormality; later in gestation, other causes, such as infection, predominate. The 1971 Swedish study[16] suggested that the role of smoking in spontaneous pregnancy termination became more severe as pregnancy progressed, but these data are difficult to interpret. It had seemed logical that smoking would have little effect on first trimester abortions or on abortions associated with chromosomal defects, but would adversely affect pregnancies in the second trimester, as it does in the third.[3]

Independently, the New York group[21] had continued to amass larger numbers in their case-control study of abortions. Their findings suggest that smoking alters the risk of trisomy and that this association varies with age. In young women aborting trisomic conceptuses, smoking was less frequent than in controls delivering at 28 weeks or later. In older women aborting trisomies, on the other hand, smoking was more common than in controls. Fitted odds ratios for smoking varied from between 0.1 and 0.5 at age 20 to between 2.0 and 3.0 at age 40 years, depending on how smoking was classified. Furthermore, the interaction between smoking and age was found to hold for different types of trisomy.

No such interaction was found for chromosomally normal aborted fetuses, although, as expected, current smoking was a risk factor (odds ratio 1.4). The New York group discussed in detail possible explanations for this unexpected interaction, including the possibility that smoking might alter the probability of a trisomic conceptus. An alternative explanation might be that smoking could alter the intrauterine survival of such a conceptus. The authors discounted artifacts arising from faulty study design or recall bias.

In a review of the effects of smoking on pregnancy outcomes, Abel[3] has enumerated a series of teratologic studies investigating the effects of nicotine on pregnancies in animals. A variety of skeletal abnormalities and fetal resorption (abortion) have been observed in chicks, mice, and pigs exposed to large doses of nicotine. Smaller doses in rats had no effect.

An accepted tenet of perinatal epidemiology is that fetal death, congenital malformation, and low birth weight often form a spectrum of effect that can result from a common cause. A fetotoxin such as thalidomide or alcohol may cause fetal death, birth defect, growth retardation, or any combination of these, depending on the period of gestation at which exposure occurred. Some of the causes of excess fetal deaths in smokers may also arise through the same mechanisms as those that lead to low birth weight or perinatal mortality. Possible mechanisms are chronic or acute oxygen deprivation resulting from increased carboxyhemoglobin levels or placental abruption or from the umbilical or amniotic infections that occur more frequently in smokers.[3] Other mechanisms by which smoking causes fetal hypoxia are decrease in placental blood flow and interference with the cellular enzymes involved in oxygen transfer. Smoking's effects may also be potentiated by marginal dietary deficiencies.

The paucity of quality research in studies of smoking and spontaneous abortion is disappointing. This lack is especially obvious when compared with the research effort that has been invested in studies of smoking and growth retardation and of pregnancy outcomes in the third trimester. Although the very real technical and logical difficulties in undertaking research on spontaneous abortions may partly explain the lack, one also senses that miscarriage is often regarded by many as a trivial event, of little public health importance.

Although many miscarriage episodes carry no serious medical or psychological consequences, a proportion certainly does. Spontaneous abortion may cause profound loss of self-esteem. Some women may suffer the financial burdens of lost earnings and excess costs for medical care. In addition, the risk of intrauterine infection is small but real, both spontaneous and arising from medical intervention to complete the pregnancy termination. Even moderate bleeding at miscarriage may lead to anemia if the woman is in a state of iron deficiency; severe bleeding may even be life-threatening. Blood transfusion carries its own risks, including an increased likelihood of maternofetal blood group incompatibility in subsequent pregnancies and the possibility of transmission of viruses such as those causing hepatitis or acquired immunodeficiency syndrome. Smokers are especially at risk for respiratory difficulties following anesthesia and are susceptible to infection and thromboembolic complications during recovery.

The complications of spontaneous abortion therefore represent a real threat to health and life for a small proportion of women in the United States. In less developed countries, this threat may be more serious. Where contraception is rare, nutrition marginal, iron deficiency widespread, and medical care unavailable or unsatisfactory, spontaneous abortion may threaten the life and health of large numbers of women. The added risk from smoking takes on special significance, therefore, in the Third World, especially in those countries where smoking among women is prevalent.

Smokers in the developed countries where research has been done experience 1.2 to 1.8 times as many spontaneous abortions as nonsmokers. In other countries, where different forms of tobacco are used and other plants are smoked, the relative risks may differ. Since the background level of spontaneous abortion is around 12% to 15% of all pregnancies,[12] the added risk to smokers means that they will have from 2.5% to 10% more miscarriages per 100 pregnancies than nonsmokers. This excess of spontaneous abortion in smokers is an unnecessary threat to life and health and a preventable burden on individual and national resources. It is one more aspect of the cost of smoking, which should be considered by governments and agencies concerned with health, prevention, and licensing and control of the tobacco industry.

REFERENCES

1. Hudson GS, Rucker MP: Spontaneous abortion. *JAMA* 1945;129:542-544.
2. Bernhard P: Die Wirkung des Rauchens auf Frau und Mutter. *Soz Med Hygiene* 1962;104:1826-1831.
3. Abel EL: Smoking during pregnancy: a review of effects on growth and development of offspring. *Hum Biol* 1980;52:593-625.
4. Zabriskie JE: Effect of cigarette smoking during pregnancy. *Obstet Gynecol* 1963;21:405-411.
5. O'Lane JM: Some fetal effects of maternal cigarette smoking. *Obstet Gynecol* 1963;22:181-184.
6. Russell CS, Taylor R, Maddison RN: Some effects of smoking in pregnancy. *J Obstet Gynaecol Br Comm* 1966;73:742-746.
7. Downing GC, Chapman WE: Smoking and pregnancy: a statistical study of 5659 patients. *Calif Med* 1966;104:187.
8. Underwood P, Hester LL, Lafitte T Jr, et al: The relationship of smoking to the outcome of pregnancy. *Am J Obstet Gynecol* 1965;91:270-276.
9. Palmgren B, Wahlen R, Wallender B: Toxemia and cigarette smoking during pregnancy. Prospective consecutive investigation of 3927 pregnancies. *Acta Obstet Gynecol* Scand 1973;52:183-185.
10. Cope I, Lancaster P, Stevens L: Smoking in pregnancy. *Med J Aust* 1973;1:73-77.
11. Stein Z., Susser M, Warburton D, et al: Spontaneous abortion as a screening device: The effect of fetal survival on the incidence of birth defects. *Am J Epidemiol* 1975;102:275-290.

12. Harlap S, Shiono PH, Ramcharan S: A life table of spontaneous abortions and the effects of age, parity and other variables, in Hook EB, Porter I (eds): *Human Embryonic and Fetal Death.* New York, Academic Press, 1980, pp 145-158.
13. Shapiro S, Levine HS, Abramovicz M: Factors associated with early and late fetal loss, in *Advances in Planned Parenthood.* VI. Proceedings of the Eighth Annual Meeting of the APPP. Amsterdam, Excerpta Medica, 1970, pp 45-63.
14. Alberman E, Elliott M, Creasy M, et al: Previous reproductive history in mothers presenting with spontaneous abortions. *Br J Obstet Gynaecol* 1975;82:366-373.
15. Kline J: An epidemiological review of the role of gravidity in spontaneous abortion. *Early Hum Dev* 1978;1:377-344.
16. Kullander S, Kallen B: A prospective study of smoking and pregnancy. *Acta Obstet Gynecol Scand* 1971;50:83-94.
17. Kline J, Stein ZA, Susser M, et al: Smoking: a risk factor for spontaneous abortion. *N Engl J Med* 1977;297:793-796.
18. Himmelberger DU, Brown BW Jr, Cohen EN: Cigarette smoking during pregnancy and the occurrence of spontaneous abortion and congenital abnormality. *Am J Epidemiol* 1978;108:470-479.
19. Hemminki K, Mutanen P, Saloniemi I: Smoking and the occurrence of malformations and spontaneous abortions: multivariate analysis. *Am J Obstet Gynecol* 1983;145:61-66.
20. Harlap S, Shiono PH: Alcohol, smoking and incidence of spontaneous abortions in the first and second trimester. *Lancet* 1980;2:173-176.
21. Kline J, Levin B, Shrout P, et al: Maternal smoking and trisomy among spontaneously aborted conceptuses. *Am J Hum Genet* 1983;35:421-431.

15 *Maternal Smoking and Weight Gain in Relation to Birth Weight and the Risk of Fetal and Infant Death*

Kenneth G. Keppel, Selma M. Taffel

The literature on smoking and reproductive health suggests that women who smoke during pregnancy gain less weight than nonsmokers; that they have relatively more fetal deaths, smaller liveborn infants, and more infant deaths than do nonsmokers; and that women who gain less weight during pregnancy have relatively more fetal deaths, smaller liveborn infants, and more infant deaths than do women who gain more weight. This paper re-examines these propositions in the light of information obtained from the

1980 National Natality Survey (NNS) and the 1980 National Fetal Mortality Survey (NFMS), conducted by the National Center for Health Statistics.

METHODS

The NNS is based on a probability sample of birth certificates of liveborn infants in the United States in the year 1980. Approximately one in 95 infants weighing less than 2500 g and one in 400 infants with higher birth weights were selected for the sample. The NFMS is based on a probability sample of reports of fetal deaths at 28 weeks of gestation or more or of infants with delivery weight of 1000 g or more in the United States for 1980.

This chapter is based on married mothers who received prenatal care (7774 in the NNS and 4699 in the NFMS). A questionnaire was mailed to the hospital named as the place of delivery on the vital record. If the medical sources failed to provide the mother's prepregnancy and predelivery weights, information supplied by the mother was used. Otherwise, the mother's prepregnancy and predelivery weights were estimated on the basis of the mother's age and race and the period of gestation. These surveys have been described in detail,[1] and a complete report on mothers' weight gain during pregnancy has been published.[2]

The National Death Index (NDI), a computerized file of information from death certificates for the United States beginning in 1979,[3] provided additional information about the deaths of infants in the NNS. Because of the relatively small number of observed infant deaths,[4] infant mortality rates based on the comparison of birth and death certificates should be interpreted with caution.

RESULTS

Smoking and Weight Gain

The average weight gain during pregnancy was 28.6 lb for smokers and 29.3 lb for nonsmokers (not significant). The only significant difference is among women who gained less than 16 lb during pregnancy: 13.6% of smokers as opposed to 9.6% of nonsmokers.

Previous studies describing an association between smoking and weight gain are based on relatively small and unrepresentative samples of women.[5,6] In the Ontario Perinatal Mortality Study, there were no differences in the weight gain distributions between smokers and nonsmokers.[7] The lack of a more definitive association between smoking and weight gain suggests that the effect of smoking on birth outcomes is not due solely to inadequate weight gain among smokers.

Smoking and Weight Gain in Relation to Risk of Fetal Death

Overall there were about 4.9 late fetal deaths per 1000 liveborn infants in 1980. The fetal death ratio for smokers was higher than for nonsmokers (5.6 *v* 4.7). This pattern was evident in all but the lowest weight gain category, although the difference was statistically significant only for mothers who gained 26 to 35 lb. Differences in the fetal death ratio with increasing maternal weight gain are more pronounced. Mothers who gained less than 16 lb had three times as many fetal deaths as those who gained 26 lb or more. The decline in fetal death ratios with increasing weight gain was evident for both smokers and nonsmokers. The probability of fetal death, measured by the life table,[8] was consistently higher for smokers than for nonsmokers for each gestation interval (Table 15-1). (However, the differences were statistically significant only for gestations of 30 to 36 weeks and 40 weeks.) This finding is consistent with that of Meyer and Tonascia,[8] who found that the probability of fetal death was higher for smokers through 36 weeks of gestation. In their study, however, the probability of fetal death was not significantly different from 36 weeks on.

Smoking and Weight Gain in Relation to Birth Weight

The mean birth weight of babies born to mothers who smoked during pregnancy was lower than that of babies born to nonsmokers by 204 g, or about 7 ounces (Table 15-2). Mean birth weight increases with maternal

Table 15-1
Probability of Fetal Death Among Married Mothers by Period of Gestation According to Mother's Smoking Habit During Pregnancy: United States, 1980 National Natality and Fetal Mortality Surveys[1]

Period of in (weeks)	Nonsmokers Probability*	Smokers Probability*	Difference in probabilities
28-29	29	36	7
30-31	34	51	17†
32-33	42	59	17†
34-35	50	63	13†
36	40	53	13†
37-39	124	126	2
40	153	199	46†
41-42	138	165	27
43	407	427	20

* Fetal deaths per 100,000 women pregnant at beginning of period of gestation.
† Significant at the .05 level for a one-tailed test.

weight gain. The mean birth weight of babies born to smokers is less than that of nonsmokers in each weight gain category; the increase in birth weight with added weight gain is evident for both smokers and nonsmokers. Additional weight gain is therefore no more beneficial for smokers than for nonsmokers. With a few exceptions, the relationships outlined above are evident when the data are controlled for period of gestation.

The literature is virtually unanimous about the adverse effect of smoking on birth weight. Most studies have found that infants born to smoking mothers weigh about 200 g less than infants born to nonsmoking mothers.[9] The association between maternal weight gain and birth weight has received less attention, but other studies have shown that inadequate weight gain is associated with smaller infants.[6,10] We found that the adverse effect of smoking on birth weight was evident in each weight gain category and that the positive effect of increased weight gain on birth weight was evident for both smokers and nonsmokers.

Smoking and Weight Gain in Relation to Infant Death

The infant mortality rate for children of smoking mothers was similar to that of nonsmoking mothers if the weight gain was less than 21 lb (21.6 and

Table 15-2
Mean Birth Beight of Live Births to Married Mothers by Weight Gain During Pregnancy, Period of Gestation and Smoking Habit of Mother: United States, 1980 National Natality Survey

Period of Gestation and Smoking Habit of Mother	Total	Weight Gain During Pregnancy (lb) <16	16-20	21-25	26-35	≥36
	Mean Birth Weight (g)					
All gestational periods						
Smokers	3236	3037	3106	3173	3266	3402
Nonsmokers	3440	3189	3266	3411	3467	3592
< 37 weeks						
Smokers	2553	2212	2343	2321	2781	2883
Nonsmokers	2715	2505	2504	2826	2846	2798
37-39 weeks						
Smokers	3153	3046	3059	3163	3157	3269
Nonsmokers	3370	3216	3277	3331	3375	3501
≥ 40 weeks						
Smokers	3414	3308	3320	3329	3428	3518
Nonsmokers	3585	3401	3420	3551	3600	3697

23.5 deaths per 1000 live births, respectively). Among women who gained 21 lb or more, however, the infants of smokers had nearly twice the death rate (11.5 and 6.6).

Findings concerning the association between smoking and perinatal mortality are contradictory. Where infant deaths are concerned, the findings depend on whether differences in birth weight are considered. It has been suggested that low weight infants born to smokers are gestationally mature while low weight infants born to nonsmokers are immature. Comparisons of mortality rates among infants weighing less than 2500 g have shown that the infants of smokers survive better.[9] All these issues cannot be resolved with the limited number of infant deaths in the NNS sample.

DISCUSSION

We began with three propositions concerning the association between smoking and infant health. These propositions have been re-examined in terms of data for married mothers from the 1980 NNS and NFMS. According to the first proposition, smokers gain less weight than nonsmokers during pregnancy. It has been suggested that the detrimental effect of smoking on birth outcomes was due primarily to inadequate weight gain among smokers.[5,6] The marginal difference in weight gain between smokers and nonsmokers observed here, and the fact that no difference was found in another major study,[7] suggest that smoking affects birth outcomes in other ways as well. Furthermore, in almost all comparisons of birth outcomes, we found that when the data were controlled for weight gain, smokers had poorer outcomes than nonsmokers.

The second proposition is that women who smoke have poorer pregnancy outcomes than those who do not smoke. This study found that mothers who smoked during pregnancy were more likely to have their pregnancy end in a fetal death or to have liveborn infants with lower birth weight and that the infants of smokers had higher infant mortality rates than those of nonsmokers. The evidence therefore indicates that mothers who smoke are at higher risk of an adverse pregnancy outcome.

The third proposition was that women who gain less weight during pregnancy have poorer pregnancy outcomes than those who gain more weight. We found that women who gained more weight had relatively fewer fetal deaths and larger liveborn infants than women who gained less weight. The association between mother's weight gain and infant's birth weight is also reflected in higher mortality rates in infants born to mothers with low weight gain.

The role of weight gain during pregnancy has not been completely explained. It is therefore not clear to what extent weight gain should be viewed as an independent variable capable of being manipulated or as a dependent variable indicative of other problems. The fact that women who gain more weight have better outcomes suggests that one strategy to improve outcomes is to encourage some women to gain more weight. Among married women in the 1980 NNS who reported that they were advised by their physicians to limit their weight gain, 27% reported a limit of 21 lb or less. Clearly, women should be given better advice about adequate weight gain. Weight gain should also be viewed as an indicator of the progress of pregnancy. However, the benefits of additional weight gain are not without limit. For example, the likelihood of a fetal death is greater for mothers with gains of 36 lb or more compared with weight gains of 26 to 35 lb. Additional weight gain improves birth outcomes for smokers and nonsmokers alike. These findings suggest that women who continue to smoke might have better outcomes with adequate weight gain. On the average, however, birth outcomes for smokers with adequate weight gain are not as good as those for nonsmokers with comparable weight gain.

REFERENCES

1. National Center for Health Statistics: *Methods and Response Characteristics: 1980 National Natality and Fetal Mortality Surveys.* Hyattsville, Md, National Center for Health Statistics. Vital and Health Statistics. Series 2, No.100: Data evaluation and methods research. US Dept of Health and Human Services publication No. (PHS) 86-1374. Washington, Government Printing Office, September, 1986.
2. National Center for Health Statistics: *Maternal Weight Gain and the Outcome of Pregnancy: United States, 1980.* Hyattsville, Md, National Center for Health Statistics. Vital and Health Statistics. Series 21, No. 44: Data from the national vital statistics system. US Dept Of Health and Human Services publication No. (PHS) 86-1922. Washington, Government Printing Office, June, 1986.
3. National Center for Health Statistics: *User's Manual: The National Death Index.* Hyattsville, Md: National Center for Health Statistics. US Dept of Health and Human Services publication No. (PHS) 81-1148, 1981.
4. Placek P, Keppel K, Coleman C, et al: Methodology for the 1980 National Natality Survey/National Death Index Match project, in *Proceedings of the Survey Research Methods Section.* American Statistical Association, Washington, 1984.
5. Rush D: Examination of the relationship between birthweight, cigarette smoking during pregnancy and maternal weight gain. *J Obstet Gynaecol Br Comm* 1974;81:746-752.
6. Davies DP, Gray OP, Ellwood PC, et al: Cigarette smoking in pregnancy: associations with maternal weight gain and fetal growth. *Lancet* 1976;1:385-387.
7. Meyer MB: How does maternal smoking affect birth weight and maternal weight gain? *Am J Obstet Gynecol* 1978;131:888-893.
8. Meyer MB, Tonascia JA: Maternal smoking, pregnancy complications, and perinatal mortality. *Am J Obstet Gynecol* 1977;128:494-502.
9. Coleman S, Piotrow PT, Rinehart W: *Tobacco—Hazards to Health and Human Reproduction.* Population Report Series L No. 1, Baltimore, Johns Hopkins University, 1979.

10. Taffel SM, Keppel KG: Implications of mother's weight gain on the outcome of pregnancy, in American Statistical Association: *1984 Proceedings of the Social Statistics Section.* Washington, 1984.

16 *Planning Status of Birth, Prenatal Care, and Maternal Smoking*

Robert H. Weller, Isaac W. Eberstein, Mohamed Bailey

The birth weight of infants born to mothers who smoke is reduced by 150 to 250 g.[1] In a pregnancy of normal duration, each cigarette smoked daily can be expected to decrease birth weight by 8-9 g.[2] Low birth weight has a number of undesirable consequences, including higher levels of neonatal and infant mortality and congenital anomalies.[3-10] The relatively poor ranking of the United States in rankings of infant mortality worldwide may be due to its unfavorable birth-weight distribution.[1,11] The rate of infant mortality could be reduced if risk factors suitable for intervention were identified.[11,12] Researchers conclude that there is "an urgent need...for research into the causes and methods of prevention of low birth weight."[13]

Evidence strongly suggests that reducing maternal smoking during pregnancy will reduce the incidence of low birth weight infants. Intervention strategies to reduce maternal smoking thus must be based on factors that influence or are associated with smoking by pregnant women. Two factors are discussed in this chapter: the pattern of prenatal care received by the mother, particularly the trimester in which she first obtains care, and whether the pregnancy is wanted or well-timed. The factors are interrelated, but each suggests an intervention point in the health care system to help reduce maternal smoking.

To investigate the role of these two factors, we evaluated the hypotheses that (1) among women who smoke before pregnancy, those who receive prenatal care early in the pregnancy (during the first trimester) are more likely than other women to stop smoking; (2) mothers with unwanted or mistimed pregnancies are more likely than other mothers to have been smokers before becoming pregnant and less likely to either stop smoking during pregnancy or to receive prenatal care early.

The idea that women who smoke at any time are more likely than other women to be smokers at any future time (including after they learn they are pregnant) and to be less likely than other women to plan their pregnancies is based on the work of Yerushalmy.[14] We expect these effects to remain valid after controlling for maternal race, education, and urban or rural county of residence, and birth order of the infant.

METHODS

Data for this research are taken from the 1980 National Natality Survey, conducted by the US National Center for Health Statistics. It is a "follow-back" survey designed to elicit detailed information about a sample of approximately 10,000 liveborn infants in the United States in 1980. Analysis is restricted to pregnancies resulting in a legitimate liveborn infant. Statistical significance means a *P*-value of .01 or less.

The hypotheses were tested by logit analysis, which uses as a dependent variable the natural logarithm of the odds of a category, where odds are computed as the ratio of the frequency of being in the category of interest to the frequency of not being in that category.[15]

RESULTS

Women who receive prenatal care in the first trimester of their pregnancies are significantly more likely than other women to stop smoking after they discover they are pregnant; obtaining early prenatal care is associated with a 2.3% increase in the probability of stopping smoking in comparison with women receiving later care or no care at all.

Women whose pregnancies are unplanned are less likely than other women to stop smoking.

Early prenatal care and having a planned pregnancy have effects on smoking behavior during pregnancy that are independent of each other, even when the control variables are introduced into analysis. Regardless of whether a woman sought prenatal care during or at some time after the first trimester, mothers whose pregnancies are unplanned (either number failures or mistimed pregnancies) are less likely than other mothers to stop smoking. Similarly, regardless of whether a pregnancy was unplanned or planned, mothers who receive early prenatal care are more likely than other mothers to stop smoking during pregnancy. All these relationships are statistically significant.

Women whose pregnancies are unplanned are less likely than other women to receive prenatal care in the first trimester; this relationship holds even after the control variables are introduced. Following Yerushalmy,[14] we had hypothesized that women whose pregnancies were unplanned would be more likely to have smoked before pregnancy. This is essentially a test of selectivity, which states that women who smoke before pregnancy are more likely than other women to have an unplanned pregnancy. If it were true, then our finding that mothers with unplanned pregnancies are more likely to continue to smoke than other women and less likely to receive prenatal care during the first trimester would be open to the suggestion that the relationship between early prenatal care and planning status of the pregnancy is spuriously produced by a common antecedent variable. For instance, Yerushalmy has argued that their unplanned pregnancies are a consequence of a lifestyle that involves more risk-taking and that they would be more likely to continue to smoke and less likely to seek early prenatal care—not because their pregnancies are unplanned but because they are risk-takers.[14] Instead, data suggest that something about having an unplanned pregnancy causes women to seek prenatal care later (if at all) and to be more likely to continue to smoke during pregnancy.

The probability that a prepregnant smoker will stop smoking after pregnancy is confirmed is .17 if she receives prenatal care during the first trimester and only .13 if she does not. In other words, obtaining prenatal care during the first trimester is associated with a 33% increase in the probability the woman will stop smoking during pregnancy. Likewise, the probability that a prepregnant smoker will stop smoking after the pregnancy is confirmed is .14 if the birth is unplanned (number or timing failure) and .17 if it is planned. Thus, wanting the pregnancy is associated with a 21% increase in the probability the woman will stop smoking during pregnancy.

Both these variables (planning status and prenatal care patterns) affect independently the probability the prepregnant smoker will stop smoking during pregnancy. Within each category of prenatal care patterns, unplanned pregnancies are associated with a lower probability that the woman will stop smoking. In each planning status category, early prenatal care is associated with a greater probability that the woman will stop smoking. By far the most interesting comparison, however, is that between the most favorable category (early prenatal care, planned pregnancy) and the least favorable category (no early prenatal care, unplanned pregnancy). In the former, the probability that the prepregnant smoker will stop smoking during pregnancy is .18, and in the latter it is only .11, a relative difference of 63%.

CONCLUSIONS

These results show that there is no selectivity involved in having an unplanned pregnancy and being a prepregnant smoker; that having an unplanned pregnancy is associated with not seeking prenatal care during the first trimester; that seeking prenatal care during the first trimester is associated with a higher likelihood the woman will stop smoking; that having an unplanne pregnancy is associated with a lower likelihood the woman will stop smok ing; and that the relationships between prenatal care and planning status and whether a pregnant woman stops smoking exist independently.

Whether a pregnancy was planned is clearly an important determinant of maternal smoking behavior during pregnancy. Mothers with unplanned pregnancies are less likely to stop smoking and, if they do not stop, smoke more than do mothers whose pregnancies are planned. This pattern remains after controls are introduced for variables such as maternal education, race, an county of residence, and birth order of the infant. Indeed, net of these factors, having an unplanned pregnancy decreases the likelihood of stopping smoking by one percentage point. Although one percentage point may not seem large in absolute terms, only 16% of prepregnant smokers stop smoking after pregnancy is confirmed. Thus a relative reduction of 6% is associated with having a planned pregnancy. Moreover, a large segment of the population is involved, with over a third of legitimate pregnancies being either number or timing failures.

Indirect effects must also be considered. A woman with an unplanned pregnancy is less likely to obtain prenatal care during the first trimester. In turn, early prenatal care is associated with an increased likelihood the mother will stop smoking. Net of maternal race, maternal education, and birth order, receiving prenatal care during the first trimester is associated with a 1.1 ercentage point increase in the likelihood the mother stopped smoking, a elative increase of almost 7%. Thus, planning status affects maternal smokng behavior in two ways. Its indirect effect is to increase the likelihood the woman will obtain early prenatal care and consequently be more likely to stop smoking. Its direct effect is independent of prenatal care.

Although the reductions in maternal smoking behavior associated with he avoidance of unplanned pregnancies may be modest, they are significant iven the strength of the relationship between maternal smoking, fetal health, irth weight, and the subsequent health of the infant. Defining a program hat could effectively reduce the incidence of unplanned pregnancies lies beond the scope of this paper. However, the importance of doing so is clear.

Only 16% of the women who smoked during the year preceding pregancy stopped smoking after pregnancy was confirmed. Even in the most faorable category, the mothers whose pregnancies were planned and who btained prenatal care during the first trimester, the probability the mother topped smoking is only .18. Why do women continue to smoke after they now they are pregnant? Why do they reduce the number of cigarettes instead f quitting altogether? Clearly the health education and health care system, as urrently structured, is insufficient to induce women to stop smoking during regnancy. Either the message is not clear enough or it is not strong enough overcome the desire (or need) of these women to continue to smoke. trategies for this type of health education and behavioral modification must e identified, evaluated, and implemented. Because prenatal care is also associated with maternal smoking behavior, a likely location for intervention is e prenatal care delivery system. However, consideration should also be iven to strategies for health education before pregnancy, which would reduce e number of unplanned pregnancies and the number of prepregnant smokers. hatever mechanisms are developed, the analysis described in this paper demnstrates the potential importance of planning status for prenatal care and marnal smoking during pregnancy, two variables closely related to pregnancy tcome.

REFERENCES

1. Brown SS: Can low birth weight be prevented? *Fam Plann Perspect* 1985;17:113-118.
2. Johnston C: Cigarette smoking and the outcome of human pregnancies: a status report on the consequences. *Clin Toxicol* 1981;18:189-209.
3. Chowdhury AKMA: Education and infant survival in rural Bangladesh. *Health Pol Ed* 1982;2:369-374.
4. Dawson I, Golden RY, Jonas EG: Birth weight by gestational age and its effect on perinatal mortality in white and in Punjabi births: experience at a district general hospital in West London 1967-1975. *Br J Obstet Gynaecol* 1982;89:896-899.
5. Federici N, Terrenato L: Biological determinants of early life mortality, in Preston SH (ed): *Biological and Social Aspects of Mortality and the Length of Life.* Liege, Belgium, Ordina Publications, 1972, pp 331-361.
6. Koops BL, Morgan LJ, Battaglia FC: Neonatal mortality risk in relation to birth weight and gestational age: update. *J Pediatr* 1982;101:969-977.
7. Levy C: Naissances hypotrophiques d'après les certificats de santé de l'anneé 1978. Leurs incidences dans la natalité: critique des données. *Population* 1982;37:945-952.
8. National Center for Health Statistics: *Adjusting Neonatal Mortality Rates for Birth Weight.* Rockville, Md, National Center for Health Statistics. Vital and Health Statistics, Series 2, No. 94, US Dept of Health, Education and Welfare publication No. (PHS) 82-1368, 1982.
9. Stewart AL, Reynolds FOR, Lipscomb AP: Outcome for infants of very low birth weight: a survey of world literature. *Lancet* 1981;1:1038-1041.
10. Taffel S: *Prenatal care, United States 1969-1975.* Rockville, Md, National Center for Health Statistics. Vital and Health Statistics, Series 21 No. 33, US Dept of Health, Education, and Welfare publication No. (PHS) 78-1911, 1978.
11. Erickson JD, Bjerkedal T: Fetal and infant mortality in Norway and the United States. *JAMA* 1982;247:987-991.
12. Peoples MD, Grimson RC, Daugherty GL: Evaluation of the effects of the North Carolina improved pregnancy outcome project. *Am J Public Health* 1984;74:544-554.
13. Lee KS, Paneth N, Gartner LM, et al: Neonatal mortality: an analysis of the recent improvement in the United States. *Am J Public Health* 1980;70:15-21.
14. Yerushalmy J: The relationship of parents' cigarette smoking to outcome of pregnancy - implication as to the problem of inferring causation from observed associations. *Am J Epidemiol* 1971;93:443-456.
15. Knoke D, Burke PS: *Log-Linear Models.* Beverly Hills, Sage Publications 1980.
16. Tienda M, Glass J: Household structure and labor force participation of black, hispanic, and white mothers. *Demography* 1985;22:381-394.

17 *Does Age Potentiate the Age-Related Risk of Perinatal Death?*

Olav Meirik, Anders Ericson, Reinhold Bergstrom

Since Simpson[1] observed the negative correlation between maternal cigarette smoking and infant birth weight, the effect of smoking on reproductive outcome has been addressed in numerous studies. Despite this research effort, a causal relationship between perinatal mortality and maternal smoking has not been established. Many authors have shown an increased risk of late fetal or early neonatal mortality in specific subgroups of mothers who had some risk factor and also smoked. Therefore maternal smoking may potentiate the adverse effect of other factors also associated with less favorable reproductive outcome.[2,3]

Increasing age of the mother is negatively related to outcome of delivery.[4,5] Cnattingius et al have recently shown that maternal cigarette smoking potentiates the age-related decrease in fetal weight gain.[6] This observation prompted us to evaluate any interactive effect of maternal age and cigarette smoking on perinatal mortality.

MATERIAL AND METHODS

In 1973 a medical birth registry (MBR) was set up in Sweden under the supervision of the National Board of Health and Welfare in Stockholm. For all births the board receives a standardized form with demographic data, previous reproductive history of the mother, and medical information about the pregnancy, the delivery, and the neonatal period. Since 1982 more data have been obtained for each birth, including the smoking habits of the mother in the first trimester of the pregnancy.

By mid-May 1985, the board had received information on 91,163 of the 92,120 births that occurred in 1983. Cases of late fetal death after 27 weeks of gestation and of early neonatal deaths were linked to the registry from death certificates. Smoking habits in the first trimester were recorded in 85,538 cases. Rates of late fetal, early neonatal, and total perinatal mortality were computed for primiparas and multiparas according to their smoking habits and age category (from 20 through 39 years). Within each age category we computed relative risks for late fetal, early neonatal, and perinatal deaths. Mothers reported to be nonsmokers served as controls in each category.

RESULTS

Maternal smoking in the first trimester was most prevalent among teen-aged mothers and decreased with increasing age (Figure 17-1). Figure 17-2 shows smoking habits among Swedish women in general, according to a survey of Swedish women conducted by the National Central Bureau of Statistics, (unpublished data, Stockholm, 1985). Teen-aged mothers tend to smoke more often than their nonpregnant peers; the reverse holds true for women later in the reproductive age-span (Figures 17-1 and 17-2).

The overall rate of late fetal death, stratified by amount of maternal smoking, is higher for smokers compared with nonsmokers, and the rate increases by number of cigarettes smoked per day (Table 17-1). This relationship also holds for perinatal deaths, but not for the early neonatal period. Late and early neonatal mortality was stratified by maternal smoking, age, and parity (Tables 17-2 and 17-3). On the whole, the rate of late fetal mortality increases by increasing age of the mother and by amount of cigarettes smoked; this relationship is most pronounced for primiparas. For early neonatal mortality, there is no clear association with either maternal age or smoking, except that light smokers appear to have a higher rate in practically all instances.

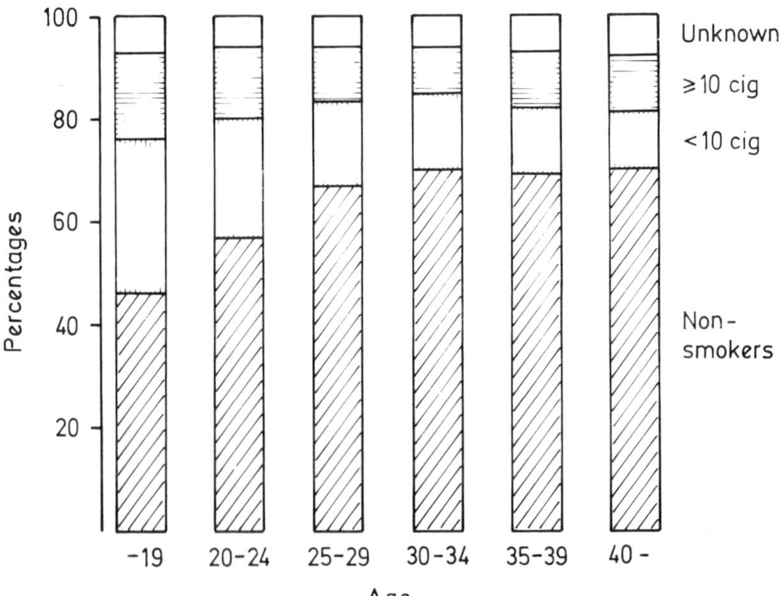

Figure 17-1 Maternal cigarette smoking by age as reported in the first trimester of pregnancy, Sweden, 1983. Percentage distribution.

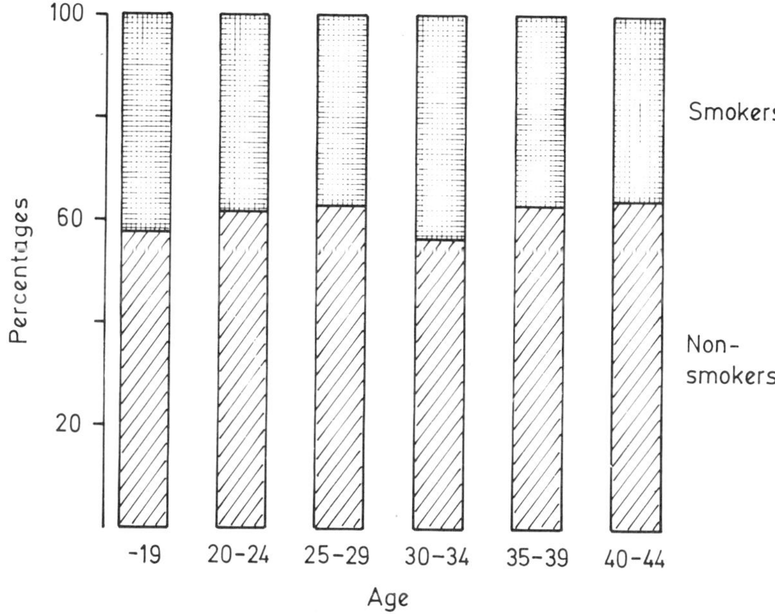

Figure 17-2 Cigarette smoking among women by age in Sweden, 1983. Percentage distribution.

The relative risks for late fetal, early neonatal, and perinatal mortality were calculated for all the age categories. Except for the ages 25-29 years, the relative risk for mortality increases with increasing amount of cigarette smoking. Mothers aged 35-39 years who smoked >10 cigarettes had significantly increased risk for late fetal and early neonatal mortality compared with non-smoking mothers of the same ages. For late fetal mortality, the relative risk increases by higher maternal age and amount of smoking, suggesting a possible interactive effect of the two factors on fetal well-being (Table 17-1).

Table 17-1
Rate per 1000 of Late Fetal, and Early Neonatal and Perinatal Mortality According to Maternal Smoking: Sweden, 1983

No. of Cigarettes	No. of Births	Late Fetal Deaths	Early Neo-natal Deaths	Perinatal Deaths
None	58,697	3.13	3.45	6.62
<10	16,243	3.32	4.57	7.88
≥10	10,598	4.25	3.70	7.93
Unknown	5,625	4.80	5.71	10.49
Total	91,163	3.40	3.82	7.21

Table 17-2
Rate per 1000 of Late Fetal Mortality According to Parity and Maternal Age and Smoking Habits: Sweden, 1983

	Age of Mother			
No. of Cigarettes	20-24 yr	25-29 yr	30-34 yr	30-39 yr
Primipara				
None	2.4 (22)	3.6 (43)	3.6 (20)	4.8 (9)
<10	3.2 (11)	3.1 (9)	4.9 (6)	8.4 (3)
≥10	5.1 (11)	3.7 (6)	6.5 (5)	6.6 (2)
Multipara				
None	1.4 (5)	2.6 (27)	3.0 (29)	3.2 (13)
<10	0.7 (1)	3.6 (10)	2.8 (6)	3.8 (3)
≥10	4.0 (4)	2.1 (4)	4.9 (7)	7.9 (5)

Numbers in parentheses denote deaths.

DISCUSSION

The results of studies dealing with maternal smoking and perinatal mortality are conflicting.[2,3,7-11] Some authors think that maternal smoking is a risk factor for perinatal mortality in high-risk populations and that in low-risk populations the effect of smoking on mortality is less.[2,11] Meyer and Comstock[2] argue that there may be populations or population subgroups in which maternal smoking is not accompanied by increased perinatal mortality. The findings from our study support their suggestion. We grouped the data by parity and age only and found that mothers in the optimal age-span for birth

Table 17-3
Rate per 1000 of Early Neonatal Mortality According to Parity and Maternal Age and Smoking Habits: Sweden, 1983

	Age of Mother			
No. of Cigarettes	20-24 yr	25-29 yr	30=-34 yr	35-39 yr
Primipara				
None	3.1 (28)	3.6 (41)	3.6 (22)	4.8 (6)
<10	4.3 (15)	4.9 (14)	4.1 (5)	2.8 (1)
≥10	5.1 (11)	1.8 (3)	5.2 (4)	19.8 (6)
Multipara				
None	3.4 (12)	3.2 (34)	3.2 (31)	2.2 (9)
<10	5.4 (8)	4.3 (12)	5.7 (12)	3.9 (3)
>10	4.0 (4)	3.2 (6)	2.8 (4)	1.6 (1)

Numbers in parentheses denote deaths.

Table 17-4
Relative Risk of Late Fetal and Early Neonatal and Perinatal Mortality for Various Age Categories According to Amount of Maternal Smoking: Sweden, 1983

No. of Cigarettes	Age of Mother			
	20-24 yr	25-29 yr	30-34 yr	35-39 yr
Late fetal deaths				
None	1.0	1.0	1.0	1.0
<10	1.1(.56,2.25)	1.1(.65,1.76)	1.2(.44,3.24)	1.4(.58,3.48)
≥10	2.2(1.19,4.06)	0.9(.77,1.05)	1.8(.89,3.61)	2.0(1.15,3.49)
Early fetal deaths				
None	1.0	1.0	1.0	1.0
<10	1.5(.88,2.43)	1.4(.88,2.16)	1.5(.85,2.53)	1.4(.46,4.16)
≥10	1.7(.96,2.96)	0.6(.28,1.26)	1.1(.46,2.36)	2.9(1.25,6.90)
Perinatal deaths				
None	1.0	1.0	1.0	1.0
<10	1.3(.86,2.35)	1.3(.88,1.87)	1.4(.83,2.32)	1.4(.70,2.83)
≥10	1.9(1.26,2.84)	0.7(.44,1.22)	1.5(.81,2.64)	2.4(1.31,4.29)

had no increased risk for perinatal mortality, but younger and older mothers had substantial risk increases.

In the older mothers we also found a tendency toward an interactive effect of age with amount of cigarettes smoked per day. The high risk as a result of heavy smoking seems to be greater for older women. In addition, young mothers (20-24 years) showed an increased risk for perinatal mortality. However, the risk factors other than smoking may be different in young and old mothers. For older mothers age itself may be the most important risk factor, which in turn is potentiated by smoking. From the data available to us we could not distinguish other risk factors or specific causes of death. Neither could we assess the independent effect of the covariating factors of age and duration of smoking prior to the index pregnancy.

Of the two components of perinatal mortality, late fetal mortality shows the most consistent association with maternal smoking in our material. Some reports have suggested that placental pathology is an important factor for fetal morbidity and mortality in pregnancies of smoking mothers.[9,12] Recently some possible pathophysiologic mechanisms by which smoking may affect fetomaternal circulation have been described.[13-16] Besides the acute effect of nicotine on maternal and placental circulation and the chronic deprivation of available oxygen by carbon monoxide, other chronic effects of smoking have recently been suggested. Severe morphologic changes in placental and umbilical vessels, which may inhibit gas exchange, have been reported by Asmussen,[13] Dadak et al,[14] Bussaca et al,[15] and Ahlsten et al[16] have found that vascular prostacyclin, which regulates vasodilation and plays an important role in blood flow maintenance, is significantly decreased in the umbilical vessels of newborns of smoking mothers. Therefore the effect of maternal smoking is probably most important in the late fetal period of the perinatal period. After birth the newborn is in fact substantially less exposed to the acute effects of maternal smoking.

Even if maternal cigarette smoking is only indirectly associated with perinatal mortality by potentiating the effect of other risk factors, such as age, the results of this study suggest that in Sweden, where maternal cigarette smoking is common, it may be the single most important preventable factor for perinatal death.

REFERENCES

1. Simpson WJA: A preliminary report on cigarette smoking and the incidence of prematurity. *Am J Obstet Gynecol* 1957;73: 808-815.
2. Meyer BM, Comstock GW: Maternal cigarette smoking and perinatal outcome. *Am J Epidemiol* 1972;96:1-10.
3. Comstock GW, Lundin FE: Parental smoking and perinatal outcome. *Am J Obstet Gynecol* 1967;98:708-718.
4. Israel SL, Deutschenberger J: Relation of the mother's age to obstetric performance. *Obstet Gynecol* 1964;24:411-417.
5. Forman RM, Meirik O, Berendes HW: Delayed childbearing in Sweden. *JAMA* 1984;22:3135-3139.
6. Cnattingius S, Axelsson O, Eklung G, et al: Smoking, maternal age and fetal growth. *Obstet Gynecol* 1985;66:449-452.
7. Underwood PB, Kesler KF, O'Lane JM, et al: Parental smoking empirically related to pregnancy outcome. *Obstet Gynecol* 1967;29:1-8.
8. Yerushalmy J: The relationship of parents' cigarette smoking to outcome of pregnancy - implications as to the problem of inferring causation from observed associations. *Am J Epidemiol* 1971;93:443-456.
9. Meyer BM, Jonas BS, Tonascia JA: Perinatal events asso- ciated with maternal smoking during pregnancy. *Am J Epidemiol* 1976;103:464-476.
10. Johnston C: Cigarette smoking and the outcome of human pregnancies: A status report on the consequences. *Clin Toxicol* 1981;18:189-209.
11. Goldstein H: Smoking in pregnancy: some notes on the statistical controversy. *Br J Prev Soc Med* 1977;31:13-17.
12. Naye RL: Effects of maternal cigarette smoking on the fetus and placenta. *Br J Obstet Gynaecol* 1978;85:732-737.
13. Asmussen I: Fetal cardiovascular system as influenced by maternal smoking. *Clin Cardiol* 1979;2:246-256.
14. Dadak C, Leithner C, Sinzinger H, et al: Diminished prostacyclin formation in umbilical arteries of babies born to women who smoke. *Lancet* 1981;1:94.
15. Bussaca M, Balconi G, Pietra A, et al: Maternal smoking and prostacyclin production by cultured endothelial cells from umbilical arteries. *Am J Obstet Gynecol* 1984;148:1127-1130.
16. Ahlsten G, Ewald U, Tuvemo T: Maternal smoking reduces prostacyclin formation in human umbilical arteries. *Acta Obstet Gynecol Scand.* In press, 1986.

18 *Smoking and Low Birth Weight: Current Concepts*

Carol J. R. Hogue, William Sappenfield

The overwhelming evidence that smoking is associated with a reduction in infant birth weight provides a strong argument for targeting smoking cessation programs for pregnant women. However, questions remain about the mechanisms by which various cigarette components retard fetal growth or trigger preterm labor. This chapter describes the relationship between maternal cigarette smoking and infant weight, as well as some postulated mechanisms of action.

Smoking behavior varies by several maternal characteristics that are also associated with low birth weight (LBW), ie, birth weight <2500 g. In illustrating those relationships, we demonstrate that the impact of smoking is fairly uniform independent of maternal characteristics, leading to a twofold risk of LBW regardless of initial maternal risk status. These risks for LBW, along with the fact that the distribution of pregnant smokers is skewed toward higher risks in general, have programmatic implications for public health practice.

EFFECT OF SMOKING ON BIRTH WEIGHT

In 1966, MacMahon et al described a uniform shift in birth weight of approximately 200 g lower weight associated with maternal smoking.[1] This reduction in birth weight has been confirmed in virtually all studies of infants of smoking mothers, including one of twins.[2] At lower birth weights, this 200 g difference can be clinically significant: there is a large difference in survival between a 1300-g and a 1500-g preterm infant. Although most infants born to smoking women are of normal birth weight, in the pregnancy sweepstakes, a woman cannot accurately predict during her pregnancy whether she will be one of the lucky ones who is gambling by smoking but eventually delivers a normal- weight infant.

The reduction in birth weight appears to be symmetrical, as there is also a reduction of crown-to-heel birth length.[3] In fact, this symmetrical growth retardation, which is related to the amount of maternal smoking in a dose-response relationship, is the most striking and consistent observation in studies of maternal smoking and infant outcome. This symmetrical growth retardation in full-term infants weighing <2500 g has been described as the "fetal tobacco syndrome" by Nieburg et al.[4] Their criteria for diagnosis of an infant with fetal tobacco syndrome include gestation > 37 weeks, ponderal index (weight in grams/length in centimeters) >2.32, no obvious cause of intrauterine growth retardation, no maternal hypertension in pregnancy, and maternal smoking of at least five cigarettes per day throughout pregnancy. The concept of a fetal tobacco syndrome has focused attention on the adverse effects of maternal smoking on infant outcome, yet it tends to underemphasize the impact of smoking by excluding many other effects associated with maternal smoking.

First, this definition excludes spontaneous abortions and preterm deliveries. Smoking is actually associated with a variety of outcomes related to fetal growth retardation throughout gestation, beginning with an increase in spontaneous abortions.[5] Smoking also increases the frequency of both preterm and full-term growth-retarded infants (Figure 18-1). At each gestational age, infants of smoking mothers had a median birth weight below those of nonsmoking mothers. Moreover, there was a dose-response relationship, with heavier smokers delivering smaller infants at each gestational age. This reduction in fetal development is primarily due to an effect on lean body mass rather than on deposition of subcutaneous fat.[6] Thus, the infant is not starving as a result of maternal smoke, but rather, the growth of the body organs is stunted.

Second, in addition to slowing fetal growth, maternal smoking increases the risk of premature rupture of fetal membranes, leading to preterm delivery,

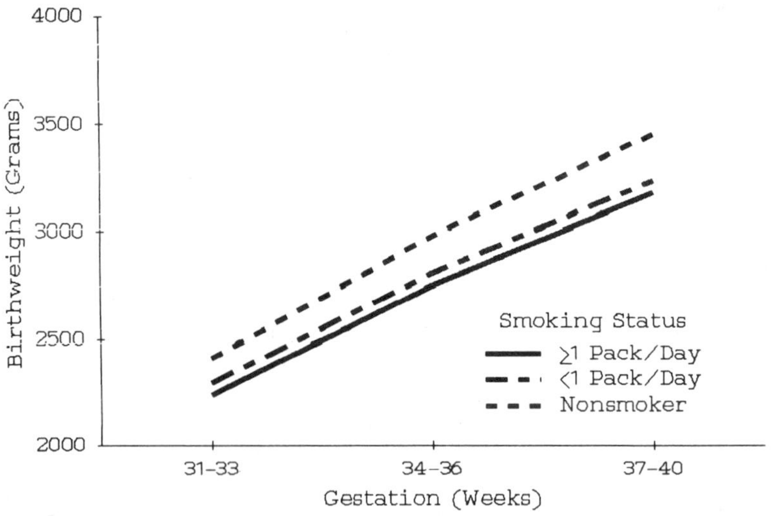

Figure 18-1 Median birth weight by maternal smoking during pregnancy for resident singleton white infants born in Missouri hospitals (Missouri birth certificate information, 1979-1981).

as well as to complications from placenta previa and abruptio placentae.[7-8] Our analysis of the 1980 National Natality Survey of white, married women revealed that 26% of the risk of preterm delivery (<36 weeks' gestation) caused by premature rupture of membranes and 39% of the risk that full-term infants will weigh <2500 g are attributable to smoking. Overall, we estimate that smoking accounts for 25% of LBW infants in the United States (Centers for Disease Control–unpublished data).

SOME POSSIBLE MECHANISMS OF ACTION

Possible mechanisms are thoroughly reviewed in the Surgeon General's report, *The Health Consequences of Smoking for Women*.[8] These mechanics include the hypoxic effects of carbon monoxide[9]; the fetal growth-retarding effects of the poisons cyanide, cadmium, and lead[10]; accelerated aging of the placenta; and maternal anemia. Why does fetal blood flow not increase to counteract the hypoxic effects of carbon monoxide? Possibly an increase in fetal blood viscosity retards fetal blood flow[11]; nicotine may also reduce the fetal blood flow.[12] There is evidence that fetal hemoglobin, hematocrit, and oxygen-hemoglobin affinity—mechanisms of acclimatization to carbon monoxide poisoning—do increase in the fetus of a smoking mother; however, this compensation is not sufficient to overcome the deficit.[13] The effect of maternal anemia has been difficult to establish, because anemia in women who smoke may go undetected. Differences in birth weight for infants of smoking and nonsmoking women with Hct values in the 41%-47% range suggest that high Hct levels in pregnant smokers may be due to a lower ratio of plasma volume to red cell mass, rather than high nutritional iron levels.[14]

One postulated "mechanism" is that smoking per se does not affect the fetus, but rather that the relationship between maternal smoking and birth weight may be a spurious one related to the type of woman who smokes.[15] That hypothesis was refuted in large part by the randomized clinical trial of Sexton and Hebel,[16] in which smokers randomly allocated to smoking cessation programs were delivered of significantly heavier infants than were smokers randomly allocated to the control group. Although a few questions remain unanswered,[17] the study strongly supports the laboratory findings that through a variety of mechanisms—some yet to be discovered—components of cigarette smoke are both fetal and maternal toxins.

SMOKERS ARE HIGHER-RISK MOTHERS

Although maternal smoking is clearly associated with lower birth weight, it is also important to recognize that smoking women are different from nonsmoking women.[15] In many respects, those differences create additional risks for the fetus. Smoking mothers are generally less educated than are nonsmoking mothers.[18,19] Smoking mothers are also younger and more often unmarried than nonsmoking mothers. Teen-agers in Missouri during 1978 were 1.6 times more likely to smoke than were women >30 years of age.[18] Unmarried women were 1.7 times more likely to smoke than were married women.[18]

Because birth certificates in Missouri include a question about smoking during pregnancy, vital records in that state are an important source of information about the relationships among maternal marital status, race, and smoking behavior during pregnancy. Between 1979 and 1981, over half of white, unmarried women smoked throughout pregnancy; in contrast, only 41.5% of black, unmarried women smoked (Table 18-1). White, unmarried women also tended to smoke more heavily; 49.5% of white smokers, compared with 19.5% of black smokers, smoked > one pack per day. For married women, there was no difference in the smoking prevalence between whites and blacks, but white married women did smoke more heavily than black married women. Because proportionately more black mothers are unmarried, the total prevalence of smoking among black mothers was higher (36.6% *v* 29.7% among white mothers). Other maternal characteristics that have also been associated with smoking include unemployment,[20] alcohol consumption, heavy coffee drinking, use of marijuana and other drugs, and nonorganic psychosis. Smoking women are also more likely not to be certain of the date of their last menstrual period,[20] which can complicate prenatal care.

INDEPENDENT EFFECTS OF SMOKING AND MATERNAL RISK STATUS

Regardless of maternal risk status, smoking women are at an increased risk of delivering an infant with LBW. In fact, the relative risk of LBW for infants of smokers compared with those of nonsmokers is approximately 2.0,

Table 18-1
Smoking During Pregnancy by Race and Marital Status, Missouri, 1979-1981

	Percentage Smoking		
	<1 pack/day	>1 pack/day	Total
Unmarried			
White	27.7	27.2	54.9
Black	33.4	8.1	41.5
Married			
White	14.5	12.6	27.1
Black	21.4	6.4	27.8
Total			
White	15.7	14.0	29.7
Black	29.1	7.5	36.6

regardless of underlying maternal risk status.[18] The combined effects of maternal risk and smoking risk appear to be multiplicatively independent. For example, a black woman with less than a high-school education who smokes exposes her infant to a nearly 20% risk of LBW; in contrast, a white woman with more than a high-school education who smokes exposes her infant to a 7.1% risk of LBW. This means that between a smoking, black woman of low education and a nonsmoking, white woman of higher education, the relative risk of delivering a LBW infant is 6.3.[18]

The finding that smoking acts as a multiplicatively independent risk factor among high-risk mothers has profound implications for public health programs focused on high-risk pregnant women. Clearly, these women should be made aware of the risks they are incurring. Smoking cessation programs should be instituted that are designed to be effective in reducing smoking among higher-risk women.

PRENATAL CARE FOR SMOKING WOMEN

The Institute of Medicine has called for an increase in smoking cessation programs designed to help pregnant women stop smoking.[21] Mass media campaigns can have an impact on nonpregnant women, pregnant women prior to their seeking care, and women under care. However, smoking cessation programs in the prenatal care setting require that women use prenatal care to benefit from them. Thus, it is important to ensure that pregnant smokers obtain prenatal care as early as possible in their pregnancies. Unfortunately, women who smoke tend to seek care later than the average woman does.18 On the other hand, some encouragement for development of effective smoking cessation interventions in prenatal care can also be seen.[18] First, in Missouri, there was an increase between 1978 and 1979-1981 in the proportion of pregnant smokers seeking care in the first trimester. Second, about three fourths of smoking women do obtain prenatal care early and are therefore available for early intervention programs.

Women who smoke during pregnancy are also less likely to receive adequate prenatal care, as indicated by the total number of prenatal care visits.[18] Again, nearly three fourths of smoking pregnant women do obtain adequate prenatal care and are thus accessible for intervention strategies.

SUMMARY

Maternal smoking has an irrefutable impact on the risk of low birth weight, as a result of both intrauterine growth retardation and an increased frequency of preterm labor. Several components of cigarettes have been found to affect either fetal growth or placental function. The risk of LBW for infants of smokers is elevated twofold over that of nonsmokers, regardless of their initial risk status. Because women who smoke tend to be at higher risk for other reasons, infants of smoking women can have as high as a one-in-four chance of being <2500 g at birth. Although smoking women tend to enter prenatal care later in gestation and to receive less adequate prenatal care than do nonsmokers, about three fourths of smoking women do receive early and adequate prenatal care. They are therefore accessible for intervention strategies for smoking cessation during pregnancy. If smoking can be stopped during pregnancy—a time when both mother and infant would benefit—it could represent a step toward a life-long health improvement that will reduce the mother's risk of premature death and enhance her child's health throughout infancy and childhood.

REFERENCES

1. MacMahon B, Alpert M, Salber EJ: Infant weight and parental smoking habits. *Am J Epidemiol* 1966;82:247-261.
2. Hemon D, Berger C, Lazar P: Maternal factors associated with small-for-dateness among twins. *Acta Genet Med Gemellol* 1982;31:241-245.
3. Persson PH, Grennert L, Gennser G, et al: A study of smoking and pregnancy with special reference to fetal growth. *Acta Obstet Gynecol Scand* 1978;78:33-39.
4. Nieburg P, Marks JS, McLaren NM, et al: The fetal tobacco syndrome. *JAMA* 1985;253:2998-2999.
5. Kline J, Stein ZA, Susser M, et al: Smoking: A risk factor for spontaneous abortion. *N Engl J Med* 1977;297:793-796.
6. Harrison GG, Branson RS, Vaucher YE: Association of maternal smoking with body composition of the newborn. *Am J Clin Nutr* 1983;38:757-762.
7. Meyer MB, Tonascia JA: Maternal smoking, pregnancy complications, and perinatal mortality. *Am J Obstet Gynecol* 1977;128:494-502.
8. US Dept of Health and Human Services: *The Health Consequences of Smoking for Women: A Report of the Surgeon General.* US Government Printing Office, 1980, pp 217-221.
9. Jouppila P, Kirkinen P, Eik-Nes S: Acute effect of maternal smoking on the human fetal blood flow. *Br J Obstet Gynaecol* 1983;90:7-10.
10. Siegers C-P, Jungblut JR, Klink F, et al: Effect of smoking on cadmium and lead concentrations in human amniotic fluid. *Toxicol Lett* 1983;19:327-331.
11. Buchan PC: Cigarette smoking in pregnancy and fetal hyperviscosity. *Br Med J* 1983;286:1315.
12. Patrick J: Fetal breathing movements. *Clin Obstet Gynecol* 1982;25:787-807.
13. Bureau MA, Shapcott D, Berthiaume Y, et al: Maternal cigarette smoking and fetal oxygen transport: A study of P50, 2,3 diphosphoglycerate, total hemoglobin, hematocrit, and type F hemoglobin in fetal blood. *Pediatrics* 1983;72:22-26.
14. Boomer AL, Christensen BL: Antepartum hematocrit, maternal smoking and birth weight. *J Reprod Med* 1982;27:385-388.
15. Yerushalmy J: The relationship of parents' cigarette smoking to outcome of pregnancy—implications as to the problem of inferring causation from observed associations. *Am J Epidemiol* 1971;93:443-456.

16. Sexton M, Hebel JR: A clinical trial of change in maternal smoking and its effect on birth weight. *JAMA* 1984;251:911-915.
17. Berman SM, Hogue CJR, Marks JS: Maternal cigarette smoking: Effect on infant birth weight, letter to the editor. *JAMA* 1985;253:1391-1392.
18. Schramm W: Smoking and pregnancy outcome. *Mo Med* 1980;77:619-626.
19. Kleinman JC, Madans JH: The effects of maternal smoking, physical stature, and educational attainment on the incidence of low birth weight. *Am J Epidemiol* 1985;121:843-855.
20. Cardozo LD, Gibb DMF, Studd JWW, et al: Social and obstetric features associated with smoking in pregnancy. *Br J Obstet Gynaecol* 1982;89:622-627.
21. Institute of Medicine. Committee to Study the Prevention of Low Birthweight. *Preventing Low Birthweight.* Washington, National Academy Press, 1985.

19 *Smoking: Prevalence, and Effects in Chile and Argentina*

Ernesto Medina, Elba Beatriz Aguirre

This chapter reviews two studies on how smoking affects birth weight in Latin America, as well as factors which influence smoking and its pathophysiologic mechanism. Although these studies are patterned after work done in the developed world, they are specific to conditions in the developing world, and may help provide insight into the tremendous public health burden of smoking-related problems.

CHILE

The prevalence of smoking, the reasons for continuing or stopping the habit during pregnancy, the relationship between cigarette smoking and birth weight, and the death risk attributable to tobacco use have been studied in Chile, a developing country. The studies were done in the capital, Santiago, which has a population of 4.5 million.

In a collaborative study of eight Latin American cities (La Plata, Argentina; Sao Paulo, Brazil; Bogota, Colombia; Santiago, Chile; Guatemala City;

Mexico City; Lima, Peru; and Caracas, Venezuela) performed under the direction of Joly et al[1,2] in 1971, 49% of men and 21% of women were found to be smokers. Roughly 10% of adult men and 5% of the women were former smokers. From these figures, it is apparent that most men and approximately 25% of the women surveyed had smoked at some time. In Santiago, 47% of the men smoked (the Latin American average[2]), but 26% of the women smoked, the highest prevalence in women in the eight cities (Figure 19-1).

From 1971 to 1984, many changes occurred in Latin America; one of the most significant areas of change was lifestyle. In Santiago, a study in 1984[3] revealed a small decrease (-6%) in men's smoking prevalence (47% to 44%) compared with the 1971 results, but an impressive increase (+50%) in women's smoking was observed, from 26% in 1979 to 39% in 1984.

In the 1984 study, the basic American Cancer Society form was used in a population survey of a random sample of 998 people. These results were applied to Santiago's census population figures to estimate the prevalence of smoking in the general population. Of women smokers, 71% smoke daily and 29% occasionally. When both sexes are averaged, the number of cigarettes smoked daily is ten. In Santiago, young people of both sexes are more likely to smoke than are the other age groups. Young women, nevertheless, are the group that smokes the fewest cigarettes daily.

Smoking During Pregnancy

Among 845 women from Santiago, we studied smoking before and during pregnancy.[4] These women did not differ significantly from the general population of Santiago in age at pregnancy, marital status, social security eligibility, educational level, illness during pregnancy, mother's weight-height index, or attitude toward pregnancy. Most had smoked at some time;

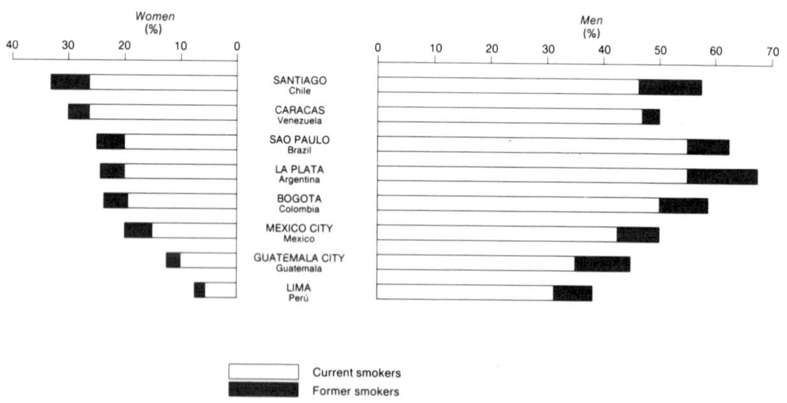

Figure 19-1 Prevalence of smoking in Latin America.

58% had smoked before pregnancy. During pregnancy, 55% of smokers stopped and 35% decreased the number of cigarettes smoked, but 11% continued smoking at the same level as before pregnancy. The reasons for mothers' changing their habit were the knowledge that smoking is harmful for the baby (49%) or nausea, vomiting, or headache (39%). Other reasons, such as the general idea that tobacco is bad for one's health, that pregnant women should not smoke, or just the lack of desire to smoke, were mentioned less frequently.

Smoking by women in Santiago varies according to age, education, marital status, and parity. There are significant differences in prevalence in the 20- to 24-year age group (65.4%) or the 25- to 29-year age group (61.4%) compared with women older than 35 years ($P < .01$). Educational level plays an important role: the prevalence of smoking in women with high-school education is higher (61%) than that observed in women with only a few years of elementary school (44%) and much higher than that in college-educated women (25%). The age-adjusted prevalence is higher in unmarried women (68%) than in married women (54%). The higher prevalence of smoking in women with low parity disappears when the data are adjusted for age. Moreover, no differences were found when pregnant women who wanted the new pregnancy were compared with those who did not.

Smoking during pregnancy among women in Santiago is associated with several factors. A high educational level, concern about the harmful effects of tobacco smoking, and having a wanted pregnancy are inversely associated with smoking during pregnancy ($P < .05$). The habit continues during gestation in women with high parity, adjusted by age, and in heavy smokers. No differences were observed according to age at pregnancy or marital status.

Birth Weight

The frequency of premature infants was twice as high in babies of smoking mothers who did not stop or decrease smoking during pregnancy than in nonsmoking women.[4] The proportion of babies with birth weight of 2500 g or less was 4.7% in nonsmoking mothers, 7.6% in those who smoked during pregnancy but decreased their consumption, and 9.6% in smoking mothers (Figure 19-2).

Infants of smoking mothers weighed an average of 220 g less than those born to nonsmoking mothers. The differences in birth weight between infants born to smokers (10 g tobacco/day) and nonsmoking women were statistically significant. These differences were also observed in the comparison of subgroups: women with or without pregnancy morbidity or women with normal or excessive weight.

The amount of birth weight deficit depends on the number of daily cigarettes during pregnancy, but it was observed even with very small daily cigarette consumption. Birth weights were similar in infants born to women who

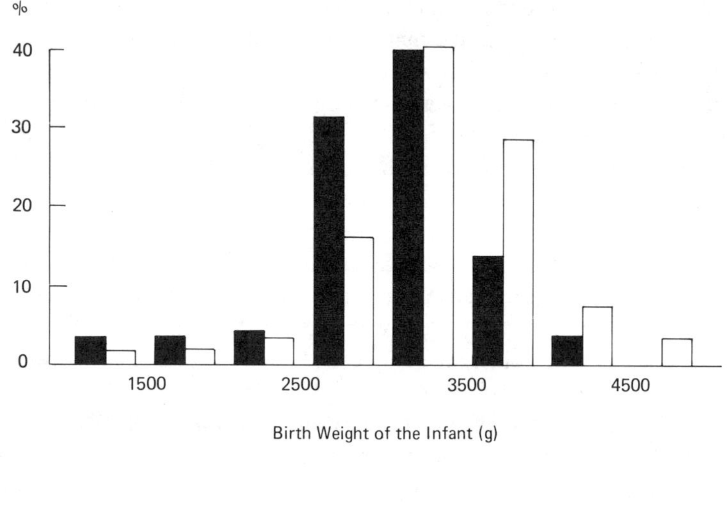

Figure 19-2 Birth weight of infants in Santiago by smoking status of the mother.

had never smoked, to former smokers who quit before pregnancy, and to women who stopped smoking during pregnancy.

Infant Mortality Attributable to Smoking During Pregnancy

In Chile, 7% of all deaths of adults are attributable to smoking; most are due to heart disease, cigarette smoking-linked malignant neoplasms, and chronic bronchitis.[3] According to the observed Chilean infant mortality rate by birth weight and the distribution of babies by the smoking status of the mother, the expected infant mortality rate in 1983 for smokers was 29.4 per 1000 liveborn infants, compared with 20.2 for nonsmoking mothers (relative risk, 1.5). With a prevalence of pregnant smokers of 26.4%, 10.2% of infant deaths are attributable to smoking.

DISCUSSION

Concern about the health effects of tobacco smoking usually appears in countries when increased life expectancy allows many people to reach old age. This implies not only a longer period of risk for addicted smokers but also a survival period of sufficient length for the pathologic conditions associated with smoking to develop. In Chile, with a life expectancy at birth of 70 years and an average cigarette consumption of 1.5 cigarettes per adult, 4543 annual deaths (7% of total adult mortality) can be directly linked to cigarette smoking, according to the attributable risk of smoking in cardiovascular diseases, malignant neoplasms, chronic bronchitis, and other diseases associated with tobacco smoking.

The information from the 1984 Santiago study survey is coincident with recent national data on cigarette production (1400 to 1500 cigarettes per adult per year). The observed prevalence of 41.2% of the adult population with an average daily consumption of ten cigarettes is equivalent to 1503 cigarettes per person per year.

The increasing prevalence of smokers in Santiago (from 36% in 1971 to 41% in 1984) and especially the upward trend observed in women are matters of concern. This tendency is associated with a relatively low level of knowledge about the harmful effects of tobacco smoking. When young women become pregnant, half of them stop smoking, but continuation by the other half causes a significant loss of birth weight and an increasing risk for babies. Unfortunately, many women who do not smoke during pregnancy resume the habit after birth, influenced by the social acceptance of smoking.

Data from tobacco smoking research lead to the conclusion that in Chile it is necessary to face very seriously the important tobacco problem we have. Strategies necessary to decrease consumption are: public education; change in the social acceptance of tobacco smoking, mainly through mass media campaigns; and an increase in cigarette prices. (A recent 50% price increase was followed by a reduction in tobacco sales of 25%.) Other important measures in Chile should be to forbid the tobacco advertisements allowed in television programs after nine o'clock at night and to maintain and increase the warning information in any type of press, radio, or television advertising.

ARGENTINA

Table 19-1 summarizes the preliminary results of a study of low birth weight among the infants of 545 pregnant women. Exposure was classified according to the average number of cigarettes smoked per day. Potentially confounding factors are not considered in the preliminary analysis. Outcome variables included residual placental blood volumes measured according to the method of Redmon et al,[5] and 47 placentas underwent pathophysiologic examination following delivery.

As the level of smoking increases, these data reflect lower birth weight, smaller cranial circumference, less residual blood in the placenta, and increased levels of perinatal mortality. These findings are similar to those of other countries but add the important finding of placentas with less blood, most likely due to small placentas among smokers. These results are preliminary, and are in the process of being expanded upon.

Table 19-1
Changes Associated with Maternal Smoking: Pirovano General Hospital, Argentina, 1984 (N=545)

Average No. Cigarettes/ Day	Birth Weight (kg)	Cranial Circum-ference (cm)	Residual Placental Blood Volume (cc)	Perinatal Mortality (%)
None	3.4	50.2	124	1.9
0-5	3.2	49.6	77	0.0
6-10	3.2	49.5	76	9.8
11-20	3.1	49.4	71	8.1
21+	3.0	49.4	66	15.1

REFERENCES

1. Joly DJ, Marchevsky N, Castilho EA, et al: Encuesta sobre las Caracteristicas del habito de fumar en America Latina. Washington, *Pan Am Health Org Sci Publ* No. 337, 1977.
2. Joly DJ, Arguelles A, Rojas F, et al: El habito de fumar cigarrillos en America Latina. Una encuesta en 8 ciudades. *Bol Of Sanit Panam* 1975;79:93-111.
3. Medina E, Pascual JP, Alegria A, et al: Tabaquismo en la poblacion general y en los medicos de Santiago, in *Actas de las IV Jornadas Chilenas de Salud Publica.* Santiago de Chile, Imprenta Valente, 1985, pp 227-229.
4. Medina E, Rojas C, Miranda R, et al: El habito de fumar de la embarazada y el peso del recien nacido. *Rev Chil Pediatr* 1984;55:279-284.
5. Redmon A, Isarra S, Ingall S: Relation of onset of respiration to placental transfusion. *Lancet* 1965;7380:283-285.

20 *Maternal Smoking and Birth Weight: An International Perspective*

Thomas T. Kane, Jason B. Smith

In numerous studies, maternal smoking has been found to be associated with low birth weight, shortened gestation, and higher rates of spontaneous abortion and perinatal mortality.[1-4] The vast majority of these studies, however, are from developed countries, and many involve relatively small study populations. These limitations mean that the relationships between smoking and adverse reproductive outcome are not as clearly established in other parts of the world and that factors of particular importance to the developing world may not have been taken into account.

For this study, a large body of data collected by Family Health International was used to examine the effects of maternal smoking on the incidence of low birth weight in a variety of cultural settings. Low birth weight is perhaps the single most important determinant of the survival chances of a newborn and a good predictor of the infant's prospects for healthy growth and development. This data set is sufficiently large to allow estimation of smoking's effects independent of other factors related to birth weight, including length of gestation, frequency of prenatal care, and maternal age and education (a proxy variable for socioeconomic status).[5-12]

METHODS

Family Health International (FHI) collects standardized information on births in more than 150 maternity centers and hospitals located in 40 countries.13 This analysis involves singleton births that occurred between 1977 and 1984 at maternity centers in seven developed and seven developing countries. The data for each country include at least 300 women who reported smoking during pregnancy. This analysis of the relationship between intensity of smoking and low birth weight includes only data sets with more than 1500 pregnant smokers. The countries represent socioeconomic and cultural settings in Asia, Latin America, and eastern and western Europe. In countries where data from more than one center were available, all the data for such countries were pooled. Centers reporting fewer than two women smoking during pregnancy were excluded from the analysis. Data were not pooled across countries because of the large variation in birth weights. The combined data sets include 95,829 women who did not smoke during the reference pregnancy and 17,813 women who smoked during all or part of the reference pregnancy. Data were analyzed by multiple regression analysis with maternal smoking during pregnancy as the primary independent variable. After additional independent variables were tested, a model was chosen that includes maternal smoking, age, education, number of antenatal visits, and duration of gestation. Maternal smoking is treated as a dichotomous variable (smoked, did not smoke during pregnancy) and as a multi-nomial variable (nonsmoker, light smoker [< one pack per day during part of pregnancy] medium smoker [> one pack per day during part of pregnancy or < one pack per day throughout pregnancy], and heavy smoker [> one pack per day throughout pregnancy]) for different parts of the analysis.

The dependent variable throughout the analysis is birth weight. In the regression analysis, birth weight is treated as a continuous dependent variable. In the cross-tabulations, two variations of the birth weight variable—mean birth weights and low birth weight—are analyzed. Low birth weight is defined as less than 2500 g.

RESULTS

Considerable variation exists in the reported prevalence of smoking among pregnant women at the various maternity centers included in this study (Table 20-1). The infants of smokers consistently had lower mean birth weights than those of nonsmokers (Table 20-2). For example, in centers in Bangladesh, Hungary, and Ireland, the unadjusted mean birth weights for infants of smokers averaged 200-300 g less than those of nonsmokers. When the data were controlled for the effects of maternal age and education, duration of gestation, and number of antenatal visits in a multiple regression model, smoking again consistently results in lower birth weight in the data sets from

Table 20-1
Number of Pregnant Women and Smoking Prevalence, by Country, 1977-1984

Country	No. of women	Percent smoking during pregnancy
Bangladesh	9,118	3.7
Brazil	11,246	20.2
Chile	16,690	25.1
Honduras	17,020	5.0
Mexico	7,443	8.8
Panama	6,859	6.4
Venezuela	13,903	23.5
Hungary	13,975	11.3
Yugoslavia	2,811	19.4
West Germany	2,011	31.7
Italy	3,716	26.1
Sweden	1,915	33.9
Austria	5,950	18.0
Ireland	985	35.7

Table 20-2
Mean Birth Weight and Difference in Birth Weights Between Infants of Smokers and Nonsmokers, by Country, 1977-1984

	Mean Birthweight (g)			
Country	Infants of Non-Smokers	Infants of Smokers	Difference (g)	Adjusted Difference (g)*
Bangladesh	2,782	2,545	-227	-147
Brazil	3,260	3,145	-115	-95
Chile	3,253	3,178	-75	-56
Honduras	3,242	3,216	-26	-27†
Mexico	3,044	3,027	-17	-32†
Panama	3,156	3,135	-21	-28†
Venezuela	3,281	3,184	-97	-92
Hungary	3,149	2,858	-291	-170
Yugoslavia	3,410	3,304	-106	-93
West Germany	3,329	3,240	-89	-63
Italy	3,316	3,217	-99	-76
Sweden	3,520	3,400	-120	-116
Austria	3,328	3,207	-121	-97
Ireland	3,601	3,380	-221	-171

* Mean birth weight of infants of smokers less than those of nonsmokers, adjusted for maternal age and education, duration of gestation, and frequency of prenatal care.
† Values are not significant at the 0.05 level.

all 14 countries. Thus, even after other important variables are held constant, the impact of smoking on birth weight is consistently negative, regardless of social or cultural setting. However, the negative coefficients of the smoking variable for the three Central American countries (Mexico, Honduras, and Panama) are not statistically significant. The net effect of smoking on birth weight after the data are adjusted for other important variables is a reduction in birth weight of between 27 g (Honduras) and 170 g (Ireland and Hungary).

The prevalence of low birth weight also varies considerably between smokers and nonsmokers in the 14 data sets (Table 20-3). About a fourth of the 8803 infants born to nonsmokers in the Bangladesh data set weighed less than 2500 g, compared with almost half (48%) of all infants born to women in Bangladesh who smoked during all or part of their pregnancies. For all countries except Honduras, smokers consistently had a higher proportion of low birth weight infants than nonsmokers. Smokers in eight of the 14 data sets had significantly higher risk of having a low birth weight infant than nonsmokers.

In the data sets with the greatest number of pregnancies during which women smoked, increasing cigarette consumption is associated with an increasing risk of delivering a low birth weight infant (Table 20-4). Heavy smokers are two to five times more likely to have low birth weight infants

Table 20-3
Percent of Birth Weights less than 2500 g and Relative Risks of Low Birth Weight, by Country and Smoking Status

	Percent of Birth Weights < 2500 g			
Country	Infants of Nonsmokers	Infants of Smokers	Relative Risks Smokers Compared with Nonsmokers	95% Confidence Intervals
Bangladesh	25.7	47.9	1.9	1.6-2.1
Brazil	4.6	7.7	1.7	1.4-2.0
Chile	7.3	8.4	1.2	1.0-1.3
Honduras	5.1	4.8	0.9	0.7-1.2
Mexico	12.1	12.8	1.1	0.9-1.3
Panama	8.6	10.4	1.2	0.9-1.5
Venezuela	6.2	7.8	1.3	1.1-1.5
Hungary	10.8	22.7	2.1	1.9-2.3
Yugoslavia	3.8	5.3	1.4	1.0-2.0
West Germany	5.4	7.5	1.4	1.0-1.9
Italy	5.5	6.0	1.1	0.9-1.4
Sweden	3.9	3.9	1.0	0.7-1.5
Austria	4.6	7.8	1.7	1.3-2.2
Ireland	2.8	6.8	2.4	1.3-4.6

Table 20-4
Relative Risks Of Low Birth Weight, by Intensity of Smoking

	Relative risks of LBW infants Smokers compared with Nonsmokers (95% Confidence Intervals)		
	*Intensity of Smoking**		
Country	Light	Medium	Heavy
Brazil	1.6 (1.2-2.1)	1.7 (1.4-2.0)	3.2 (1.4-6.3)
Chile	1.2 (1.0-1.3)	1.1 (0.9-1.3)	2.9 (1.1-5.8)
Venezuela	1.1 (0.9-1.3)	1.4 (1.2-1.7)	2.4 (1.0-4.7)
Hungary	1.8 (1.6-2.1)	2.3 (2.0-2.6)	5.0 (3.2-6.7)

* Light smoking = < one pack/d; medium smoking = > one pack/d for part of pregnancy or < 1 pack/d throughout pregnancy; heavy smoking = > 1 pack/d throughout pregnancy.

than nonsmokers. This evidence corroborates the findings of earlier studies that the effect of smoking on birth weight is dose-related.[4,8]

DISCUSSION

These data are consistent with those of studies from other countries in showing a consistent pattern of increased risk of low birth weight according to whether and how much a mother smokes during pregnancy. This relationship is found regardless of country, maternal age and education, the number of antenatal visits, or duration of gestation.

How smoking affects birth weight remains unclear. Several components of smoking and tobacco may play a role, but the most likely explanation is increased blood levels of carbon monoxide and consequent reduction in the oxygen-carrying ability of hemoglobin supplying the fetus.[14-17] Nicotine is also thought to reduce placental blood flow because of its vasoconstriction of blood vessels.[3,14] Vitamin depletion due to cyanide and maternal appetite suppression are also possibilities.[3] Some researchers contend that low birth weight is the result of self-selection of the smokers rather than smoking itself.[18-20] Poor women may tend to smoke more but also may have more health problems and poorer nutritional status than women of higher socioeconomic status. However, this argument is inconsistent with the results of this and other studies that show evidence of a dose-response relationship between smoking and birth weight, as well as with those of studies that reflect lower birth weight during pregnancies when a woman smokes compared with pregnancies of the same woman when she did not smoke.[21-23]

Data in this analysis relate to deliveries in selected hospitals and maternity centers and do not include information on the large proportion of births that occur at home in many developing countries. Mean birth weights among home deliveries may differ from those among hospital births. Smoking behavior may also vary between women delivering at home and at hospitals. The socioeconomic and health status of women and the average birth weight of their children may also vary between hospitals in each country as well as between countries.

These data are not representative of all births in the countries where the maternity centers are located or even of hospital births in those countries. The maternity centers and hospital included in this analysis are self-selected. Some centers may serve mostly women of higher socioeconomic status in urban areas; others may serve predominantly poor, unhealthy women in rural areas of the same country. Data from maternity centers within each country were pooled, primarily to obtain enough smokers without having to pool data from different countries, which would cause even wider variations in birth weights, client characteristics, medical facilities, and health conditions.

Some potential sources of bias in these data should be considered. The overall prevalence and intensity of smoking may have been underreported. Because smoking is still viewed as socially unacceptable behavior for women in many countries (especially for pregnant women), some women who smoke during pregnancy may not report it. Underreporting of smoking would result in some births to smoking women being included with the data for nonsmoking women. If the birth weights of infants of smoking women are lower than those of infants of nonsmoking women, then the inclusion of some infants of smoking women with the infants of nonsmokers would tend to lower the mean birth weight for infants of nonsmokers and increase the proportion of infants under 2500 g born to nonsmokers. This would result in an underestimation of the difference in birth weights between smokers and nonsmokers.

Since the vast majority of births in developed countries occur in hospitals, birth weight data are less likely to be affected by selection bias in those countries. In developing countries, however, birth weights may be higher or lower for hospital deliveries compared with home deliveries. Hospital births in developing countries often include a higher proportion of births with pregnancy and delivery complications. On the other hand, women delivering in hospitals in developing countries may be of higher socioeconomic status and in better health and therefore give birth to heavier babies than the majority of women, who deliver at home.

The birth weight data collected from the maternity centers included in this analysis are accurate to the nearest 10 g. The data sets from some of the developing countries show strong evidence of a disproportionately high number of birth weights at even 100-g intervals. For example, there is a great deal of clustering in the birth weight data from the Bangladesh maternity centers, but the Hungary data set has very little. Heaping of birth weights does not seriously bias the results, although it will affect the precision of the estimates.

There may be considerable variation in the data quality from the different maternity centers. Some centers have very motivated and trained staff with good research skills and data collection experience (such as university teaching hospitals); other centers have very few trained staff and limited resources. The data quality and the data collection instruments (the Maternity Record Form) have been described in detail elsewhere.[9,13]

A number of variables have been identified as risk factors for low birth weight. We have examined some of them, including maternal smoking, age, education, duration of gestation, frequency of prenatal care, and nationality. Many other factors may be controlled for in the analysis of the effects of smoking on birth weight. Other potentially important risk factors are maternal height and prepregnancy weight, race/ethnic origin, marital status, parity, selected diseases such as diabetes, malaria, and chronic hypertension, selected infections such as rubella and chlamydia, poor nutritional status, anemia, toxemia, alcohol and drug abuse, previous pregnancy and obstetric history, fetal anomalies, length of interpregnancy interval, multiple pregnancy, sex of fetus/infant, placental problems during pregnancy (such as placenta previa), and maternal genetic factors such as low maternal weight at own birth.[12]

Birth weight also varies according to altitude and season in some countries.[4,12,14] These may also be important control variables for a mountainous country such as Chile (altitude factor) or a country that experiences dramatic seasonal or annual fluctuations in food supply, such as Bangladesh (seasonal factor).

Maternal nutritional deficiencies and infectious and parasitic diseases are likely to play a much larger role in determining birth weights in many developing countries. These factors may act to compound or obscure the effects of smoking on birth weight in these areas.

The effects on pregnant women who do not smoke but live or work in an environment where they are exposed to the smoke of others are not addressed in this analysis but may be important. It is also beyond the scope of this analysis to evaluate the impact of other uses of tobacco by pregnant women (such as pipe or cigar smoking, tobacco chewing, or use of snuff) on birth weight.

CONCLUSION

The evidence in this study is consistent and clear for both developed and developing countries alike. Smoking is related to the risk of low birth weight in every country examined. It would be useful to extend the analysis to see how smoking and low birth weight are linked to prematurity and perinatal mortality. More research needs to done on the effects of maternal smoking on birth weights in developing countries. The World Health Organization recently reported that cigarette smoking has been increasing in developing countries at an annual rate of 2.1%. This translates into a doubling of the smoking population in one generation (33 years). The evidence from all 14 data sets (including seven from developing countries) consistently show that maternal smoking is associated with lower birth weight, even after other important variables are controlled.

Public health intervention and educational programs should continue to be developed and intensified worldwide to discourage women from smoking during pregnancy. In developing countries where the incidence of low birth weight deliveries is already high, any increase in the prevalence of smoking among pregnant women will aggravate this problem.

Reducing smoking during pregnancy will undoubtedly help to reduce the incidence of low birth weight and the inherent high health risks and costs that often accompany such births.

Acknowledgments

The authors appreciate the help of Peter Myers, Kim Sterling, Lynne Wilkens, Gary Grubb, Michael Rosenberg, Barbara Janowitz, and Jim Higgins.

REFERENCES

1. Abel EL: *Smoking and Reproduction: An Annotated Bibliography.* Boca Raton, Florida, CRC Press, Inc, 1984.
2. Tudehope DS, Sinclair JC: Birthweight, gestational age, and neonatal risks, in Behrman RE (ed), Driscoll JM, Seeds AE (assoc eds): *Neonatal Perinatal Medicine: Diseases of the Fetus and Infant.* St. Louis, CV Mosby Co, 1977, pp 116-127.
3. Coleman S, Piotrow PT, Rinehart W: *Tobacco—Hazards to Health and Human Reproduction.* Population Reports, series L, No 1. Population Information Program. Baltimore, Johns Hopkins University, 1979.
4. Fried PA, Oxorn H: *Smoking for Two: Cigarettes and Pregnancy.* New York, The Free Press, 1980.
5. Dougherty CRS, Jones AD: The determinants of birthweight. *Am J Obstet Gynecol* 1982;144:190-200.
6. Gould J: Maternal smoking affects birthweight regardless of social class. *Birth* 1984;11:229.
7. Kleinman JC, Madans JH: The effects of maternal smoking, physical stature, and educational attainment on the incidence of low birthweight. *Am J Epidemiol* 1985;121:843-855.
8. Meyer MB, Jones B, Tonascia JA: Perinatal events associated with maternal smoking during pregnancy. *Am J Epidemiol* 1976;103:464-476.
9. Potts M, Janowitz BS, Fortney JA (eds): *Childbirth in Developing Countries.* Boston, MTM Press, 1983.
10. Wainright RL: Change in observed birthweight associated with change in maternal cigarette smoking. *Am J Epidemiol* 1983:117:668-675.
11. World Health Organization: The incidence of low birthweight: A critical review of available information. *World Health Stat Q* 1980;33:197-224.
12. Committee to Study the Prevention of Low Birthweight, Behrman RE, Chairman, Division of Health Promotion and Disease Prevention, Institute of Medicine: *Preventing Low Birthweight.* Washington, National Academy Press, 1985.
13. Janowitz B, Lewis J, Burton N, et al: *Reproductive Health in Africa: Issues and Options.* Research Triangle Park, NC, Family Health International, 1984.
14. Naeye RL, Tafori N: *Risk Factors in Pregnancy and Diseases of the Fetus and Newborn.* Baltimore, Williams & Wilkens Co, 1983.
15. D'Souza SW, Black PM, Williams N, et al: Effect of smoking during pregnancy upon the haematological valves of cord blood. *Br J Obstet Gynaecol* 1978;85:495-499.
16. Garn SM, Shaw HA, McCabe KD: Effect of maternal smoking on hemoglobins and hematocrits of the newborn. *Am J Clin Nutr* 1978;31:557-558.
17. Longo LD: The biological effects of carbon monoxide on the pregnant woman, fetus, and newborn infant. *Am J Obstet Gynecol* 1977;129:69-103.

18. Silverman DT: Maternal smoking and birthweight. *Am J Epidemiol* 1977;105:513-521.
19. Yerushalmy J: Infants with low birthweight born before their mothers started to smoke cigarettes. *Am J Obstet Gynecol* 1972;112:277-284.
20. Hickey RJ, Clelland RC, Bowers EJ: Maternal smoking, birthweight, infant death, and the self-selection problem. *Am J Obstet Gynecol* 1978;13:805-811.
21. Murphy JF, Mulcahy R: The effect of age, parity, and cigarette smoking on baby weight. *Am J Obstet Gynecol* 1971;111:22-25.
22. Savel LE, Roth E: Effects of smoking in pregnancy: a continuing retrospective study. *Obstet Gynecol* 1962;20:313-316.
23. Underwood P, Hester LL, Gregg KV: The relationship of smoking to the outcome of pregnancy. *Am J Obstet Gynecol* 1965;91:270-276.

21 *Effect of Tar, Nicotine, and Carbon Monoxide on Pregnancy Outcome*

Sherrie Aitken, Robert Laforge, Danielle Spiegler, Paul Placek, Henry Malin

Much remains unknown about the relationships among smoking, drinking, and pregnancy outcomes. For example, we do not know how cigarette types influence the level of exposure to the constituents in cigarettes, nor do we know which component of cigarettes—tar, nicotine, or carbon monoxide—is linked to low birth weight. We do not know whether smoking is more harmful during the early or later stages of pregnancy. Finally, we do not know how stopping or switching to less potent cigarettes during pregnancy affects the risk of low birth weight.

In most studies of the association between smoking and low birth weight, the number of cigarettes smoked has been measured without consideration of the fact that brand and other cigarette characteristics cause wide variations in the amounts of toxins in each.[1,2] This analysis examines the risk for low birth weight posed by differing average daily exposures to tar, nicotine, and carbon monoxide, as well as number of cigarettes. Average daily exposure to cigarette toxins was hypothesized to be a more sensitive measure than number of cigarettes alone.

Since many smoking mothers reduce or stop smoking after pregnancy is confirmed,[3-7] this paper examines the possibility that different levels of cigarette toxin exposure before and after confirmation of pregnancy might differentially affect the risk of low birth weight.

METHODS

This analysis is based on the 1980 National Natality Survey (NNS), conducted by the National Center for Health Statistics. The 1980 NNS was a mailed follow-back survey of mothers, hospitals, and other medical sources identified on birth certificates for 9941 liveborn infants.[8] Low birth weight infants were oversampled to support detailed analyses of high-risk infants. Information from the birth certificate was linked to the questionnaire mailed to each married mother, which requested information about prenatal health practices, such as drinking and smoking, prenatal medical visits, and other demographic characteristics. This analysis includes 3751 white married mothers of singleton infants, among them 1116 smokers for whom cigarette component values could be derived.

Exposure to cigarette components was grouped into four levels and examined for three time periods (before, after, and throughout pregnancy). Multiple logistic regression provided estimates of risk after the data were controlled for the mother's age, education, height, prepregnancy weight, weight gain during pregnancy, number of prenatal visits, history of miscarriages, stillbirths or abortions, and alcohol use. The model also controlled for birth order, gestation period, sex of infant, and father's height. A forced multiple logistic regression model was employed which allowed risk comparison of different levels of cigarette exposure against the reference group of nonsmokers.[9] In all the regressions evaluating cigarette toxins, our model provided a good fit to the predicted model, as determined by Hosmer's goodness-of-fit statistics.[10]

Cigarettes low in one component tend also to be low in others; the correlation among tar, nicotine, and carbon monoxide content was 0.86. Because of this relationship, the independent effects of tar, nicotine, and carbon monoxide could not be separated. Tar, nicotine, and carbon monoxide content were taken from reported cigarette characteristics.[2] Tar, nicotine, and carbon monoxide values were multiplied by the number of cigarettes smoked daily to estimate average daily exposures.

Exposure levels were derived from the quartile distribution of average daily exposure to cigarette toxins for the 922 smokers who did not stop smoking during pregnancy. Hence, each exposure level contained approximately one quarter of the smokers who did not quit. Risk of low birth weight was estimated for each level of exposure compared with that among nonsmokers. Mothers who quit smoking after pregnancy was confirmed were analyzed separately, so that their data did not contribute to the calculation of the cigarette toxin levels or risk estimates for smokers who continued to smoke.

To examine the effect of reducing smoking during pregnancy, risk of low birth weight was determined for the period after conception but before pregnancy was confirmed, for the period after pregnancy was confirmed, and for both periods combined ("before," "after," and "throughout" pregnancy).

RESULTS

Thirty percent (1116) of the women in this sample smoked at the time of conception. After pregnancy was confirmed, 5% (194) stopped smoking; 25% (922) smoked throughout pregnancy. Most smokers (93%) did not change cigarette brands during pregnancy. Smokers who switched brands tended to change to less potent cigarettes. These brand-switchers experienced a risk of low birth weight higher than that of nonsmokers, but not significantly so (relative risk [RR]=1.8, 95% confidence interval [CI] 0.8-4.0).

Mean daily exposure to tar, nicotine, and carbon monoxide decreased after pregnancy was confirmed because women either reduced the number of cigarettes smoked or switched to less potent cigarettes. Average daily exposure was higher during the "before" period and lower during the "after" period. Since the "throughout" pregnancy period is a composite of these two periods, the average daily exposure levels for "throughout" fall between those of the other two periods.

Quitters:

Mothers who quit smoking after pregnancy was confirmed tended to be lighter smokers than those who did not. The adjusted relative risk for smokers who quit was 1.1, not significantly different from that of nonsmokers.

Adjusted estimates of risk of low birth weight were calculated by cigarette toxin exposure levels for the three time periods (Table 21-1). These estimates represent the odds ratio for low birth weight attributable to cigarette toxin exposure after the data were adjusted for potentially confounding factors.

A dose-response relationship between exposure to cigarette toxins and relative risk of low birth weight was found at all but the lowest level of exposure. The risk of low birth weight among smokers in the highest exposure groups was over three times that of nonsmokers.

Impact of Before/After Exposure:

Only small and inconsistent differences in the risk of low birth weight were found between the "before" and "after" time periods, indicating that cigarette exposure before pregnancy is confirmed does not differ in its risk of low birth weight from exposure later in pregnancy.

Table 21-1
Adjusted Risk of Low Birth Weight by Cigarette Toxin Exposure Levels: Married Mothers of Live Single Births in the 1980 National Natality Survey

	Relative Risk of Low Birth Weight (N=922)		
Exposure	Before Pregnancy	After Pregnancy	Throughout Entire Pregnancy
Tar Level			
1 (low)	1.1*	1.4*	1.2*
2	2.0	1.9	2.1
3	2.4	2.7	2.7
4 (high)	4.1	3.3	3.3
Nicotine Level			
1 (low)	1.3*	1.4*	1.2*
2	1.5*	2.0	2.0
3	2.8	2.5	2.8
4 (high)	3.8	3.3	3.2
Carbon Monoxide Level			
1 (low)	1.1*	1.3*	1.1*
2	1.8	2.0	2.1
3	2.6	2.3	2.5
4 (high)	3.9	3.7	3.8

* All relative risk values are significant at the .05 level or less except those noted with an asterisk.

Characteristics of Quitters:

The risk for mothers who stopped smoking during pregnancy compared with nonsmokers was 1.1, which is not significant. In other words, mothers who quit were no more likely to have a low birth weight infant than were mothers who had no previous history of smoking. This result might be partially due to selection differences, since mothers who stopped smoking tended to have been lighter smokers than those who did not. Over half the mothers who stopped smoking after pregnancy was confirmed smoked fewer than ten cigarettes a day; only a fourth of the smokers who did not quit smoked at or below that level. In addition, educational attainment is directly related to the tendency to quit smoking during pregnancy. This finding was also reported by Prager et al.[7]

Correlation of Toxin Measures:

A comparison of cigarette toxin measures with number of cigarettes found little difference between the measures. The correlation of the measures

Table 21-2
Risk of Low Birth Weight for Selected Maternal and Infant Characteristics: All White Married Women of Live Single Birth Infants in the 1980 National Natality Survey

Independent Variable	Odds Ratio	Referent Group
Tar (throughout pregnancy) (M)		
1st (lowest) exposure level	1.2*	
2nd quartile exposure level	2.1	
3rd quartile exposure level	2.7	Nonsmokers
4th (highest) exposure level	3.3	
Smokers who quit	1.1*	Nonsmokers
Female sex	1.5	Male
Weight Gain of < 20 lb	2.0	> 21 lb
Educational Attainment < 12 yr	1.0*	12+ yr
Mothers aged ≥ 35 yr	2.0	< 35 yr
Prepregnancy weight < 130 lb	1.7	> 131 lb
Mothers height < 63 in	1.8	> 67 in
Mothers height 63-66 in	1.1*	
Fathers height < 69 in	1.0*	> 73 in
Fathers height 69-72 in	1.1*	
Period of gestation < 37 wk	30.7	> 37 wk
Livebirth order first child	1.3	2nd or greater
Number of prenatal visits < 5	3.8	> 5
Any previous miscarriages, stillbirths, or abortions	1.3*	None
Average daily ethanol consumption (oz daily)	1.5	Nondrinkers

Low birth weight is defined as less than 2500 g.
* *P*-value > .05.

of average daily tar, nicotine, and carbon monoxide with number of cigarettes smoked per day is 0.76.

The correlation coefficients of birth weight with measures of the number of cigarettes per day and average daily exposure to cigarette toxins were calculated for the three time periods. Although small differences in the correlation coefficients were found, none reached statistical significance at the .05 level. In addition, a dose-response relationship on the same order of magnitude as that for exposure to cigarette toxins (Table 21-1) was found for number of cigarettes and relative risk of low birth weight (data not shown). This dose-response relationship suggests that, at least for this sample of smokers, measures of the number of cigarettes are as good a predictor of low birth weight as are the measures of strength of cigarette toxins.

Sex of the infant; mother's weight gain, age, height, and prepregnancy weight; period of gestation; birth order; number of prenatal visits; and alcohol consumption were all independently associated with significantly increased risk of low birth weight (Table 21-2). The range of the relative risk estimates for these risk factors are comparable with those reported in other studies of low birth weight.[11,12]

DISCUSSION

This analysis demonstrates a dose-response relationship of exposure to cigarette toxins with relative risk of low birth weight among white married mothers of liveborn single-birth infants. An increased risk of low birth weight was found for women who reported smoking as few as seven cigarettes per day. The estimates of relative risk increased directly with exposure to cigarette toxins above this level, and typically the relative risk was even greater after the data were adjusted for a variety of known risk factors for low birth weight. Although separate effects of tar, nicotine, or carbon monoxide could not be demonstrated with these data, these findings provide evidence that cigarette exposure, measured either in milligrams of cigarette toxin per day or in number of cigarettes smoked per day, is an important risk factor for low birth weight. Measures that account for the potency of cigarette toxins were not found to be better predictors of low birth weight than are simple counts of the number of cigarettes smoked.

A further complication is raised by several recent studies in which smokers of low-yield cigarettes were found to have about the same plasma nicotine and carbon monoxide levels as those who smoke regular brands.[13,14] Smokers of low-yield cigarettes may "compensate for reduced yields by altering their smoking methods, so that the amounts of tar and nicotine they receive may actually bear little relation to reported yields."[15] The findings for smokers who switched brands after pregnancy was confirmed also indicate that it may be important to measure the potency of cigarette toxins. Finally, the failure to detect a difference between these measures may be due to other biases introduced in the method of data collection. Since women were contacted 3 to 7 months after delivery and asked to recall their smoking behavior, this imprecision may have affected the results.

Smokers tended to reduce their smoking after pregnancy was confirmed. This finding is consistent with the reduction in cigarette consumption reported for the entire 1980 NNS sample[7] and in other studies.[4,6] Despite this reduction, no evidence was found that smoking early in pregnancy is more harmful than in later pregnancy. However, since our analysis did not control for the confounding effects of exposure over time, these findings should be viewed with caution.

Mothers who quit smoking after pregnancy was confirmed were no more likely to have low birth weight infants than were nonsmoking mothers. This finding has important practical implications for prevention policy. Hence, it should not be dismissed outright because of the selection questions. At the least, this finding suggests that smokers who quit may lower their risk of delivering a low birth weight infant and should be the subject of further research. This view is supported by a recent clinical trial in which fetal growth retardation was found to be overcome by providing antismoking assistance to pregnant smokers.[5]

REFERENCES

1. US Dept of Health and Human Services: *The Health Consequences of Smoking for Women: A Report of the Surgeon General.* Government Printing Office, 1980, pp 189-250, 336-349.
2. Federal Trade Commission: How do your cigarettes stack up for tar, nicotine and carbon monoxide? March 1981.
3. Prager K, Malin H, Graves C, et al: Maternal smoking and drinking before and during pregnancy, in *Health United States 1983.* US Dept of Health and Human Services publication No. (PHS) 84-1232, National Center for Health Statistics. Government Printing Office, December 1983.
4. Kuzma SW, Kissinger DG:. Patterns of alcohol and cigarette use in pregnancy. *Neurobehav Toxicol Teratol* 1981;3:211-221.
5. Sexton M, Hebel JR: A clinical trial of change in maternal smoking and its effect on birthweight. *JAMA* 1984;25:911-915.
6. Wilner S, Schoenbaum SC, Palmer RH, et al: *Smoking and Quitting Drinking During Pregnancy: Who Does and Who Doesn't.* Institute for Health Policy Studies, University of California, San Francisco, January 1985 (unpublished).
7. Prager K, Malin H, Spiegler D, et al: Smoking and drinking behavior before and during pregnancy of married mothers of live-born infants and still-born infants. *Public Health Rep* 1984;99:117-127.
8. Placek PJ: The 1980 National Natality Survey and National Fetal Mortality Survey—methods used and PHS agency participation. *Public Health Rep* 1984;99:111-116.
9. Lemshow S, Hosmer D: Estimating odds ratios with categorically scaled covariates in multiple logistic regression analysis. *Am J Epidemiol* 1984;119:147-151.
10. Dixon VJ (ed): *BMDP Statistical Software: 1985 Printing,* Berkeley, Calif, University of California Press, 1985.
11. Taffel SM, Keppel KG: Implications of mother's weight gain on the outcome of pregnancy. Proceedings of the American Statistical Association Social Sciences Section, Winter 1984-1985 (unpublished).
12. Mills JL, Graubard BI, Harley EE: Maternal alcohol consumption and birthweight: How much drinking during pregnancy is safe? *JAMA* 1984;252:1875-1879.
13. Benowitz NL, Hall SM, Herning RI, et al: Smokers of low-yield cigarettes do not consume less nicotine. *N Engl J Med* 1983;309:139-142.
14. Hoffman D, Adams JD, Haley NJ: Reported cigarette smoke values: a closer look. *Am J Public Health* 1983;73:1050-1053.
15. Fielding JE: Smoking: Health effects and control. *N Engl J Med* 1985;313:555-561.

22 *Maternal Smoking Trends in Missouri*

Garland H. Land, Joseph W. Stockbauer

Since 1978, birth and fetal death certificates in Missouri have included a question about the amount of cigarettes smoked by the mother during pregnancy per day. Missouri thus has one of the largest population-based databases for smoking during pregnancy in the world. A comparison of this database with the 1980 National Natality Survey (NNS) illustrates maternal smoking trends since 1978 and identifies populations at high risk for smoking which can be targeted for intervention or cessation efforts.

The 1980 NNS and 1980 Missouri data for married women are similar (Table 22-1). The NNS-based estimate of smoking prevalence during pregnancy for the United States in 1980 was 26.3%, compared with 27.3% of Missouri women. Both data sets show that married mothers who smoke during pregnancy are most likely to be white, under age 25 years, and with less than 12 years of education. Of the Missouri women, 2.9% started prenatal care in the third trimester while 3.7% of the NNS women did, otherwise most demographic characteristics measured in both the NNS and Missouri data agree to within two standard errors of the NNS estimate. Larger differences for nonwhites, older women, and less educated women possibly reflect problems with a lower response rate in the NNS. Information on maternal smoking is available from the birth certificate for 99.6% of births in Missouri; in contrast, the response rate for the smoking question on the NNS is only 56%.

Since the NNS does not include data on single mothers, the Missouri data can provide a more complete picture of all women who smoke during pregnancy. Single mothers who smoke, like married smokers, tend to be white and less educated. However, older single smoking mothers have higher smoking rates than the younger ones; the opposite is true for married mothers. When data for married and unmarried women are combined, the distribution of births by mother's age and education is very similar to that of the married population, since most of the mothers are married. However, the percent of smoking mothers by racial category is reversed. For all births more nonwhites smoke (35.3%) than whites (30.0%)(Table 22-1), which is a reversal of the separate findings for married and unmarried women. This mainly reflects the higher smoking rates among the unmarried population.

The Missouri data allow comparison of smoking trends since 1978 among pregnant women. Between 1978 and 1984, the proportion of women who smoked during pregnancy dropped slightly. During this 7-year span, the

Table 22-1
Mothers of Liveborn Infants Who Smoked During Pregnancy, Missouri and United States, 1980

	1980 US National Natality Survey (%)	1980 Mo. Married (%)	1980 Mo. Not Married (%)	1980 Mo. Total (%)
All mothers	26.3	27.3	47.4	30.8
Race				
White	27.0	27.4	54.9	30.0
Nonwhite	20.9	25.9*	41.4	35.3
Mother's Age (yr)				
<20	40.0	41.1	42.4	41.7
20-24	31.8	31.2	51.7	34.9
25-29	21.3	21.2	50.2	23.6
30-34	19.2	22.1*	49.2	23.9
35+	20.8	25.4*	57.4	28.0
Education (yr)				
<12	43.8	51.5*	52.9	52.0
12	28.1	27.6	43.9	29.9
13-15	20.1	18.0*	36.9	20.1
16+	10.3	9.8	22.1	10.0

1980 NNS information represents weighted national estimates of maternal smoking during pregnancy; data were produced by the Natality Statistics Branch, Division of Vital Statistics, NCHS.
*As compared with NNS, $P<.05$.

proportion of smokers dropped nearly 15% in nonwhite women but only 5% among white women. With this larger drop among nonwhites, the smoking rates in 1984 were similar for nonwhites and whites. Pregnant women with the highest smoking rates in the late 1970s were nonwhites, teen-agers, singles, those with less than 12 years of education, and those with three or more children. The smoking pattern in the mid-1980s shows two substantial changes. Smoking rates for nonwhites are now only slightly higher than those of whites, and smoking rates for teen-agers, while still high, are about the same as those of the 20-24 age group. It is encouraging that the groups with the poorest reproductive outcomes and the highest smoking rates in the past (nonwhites and teen-agers) are showing the greatest decreases in smoking rates during pregnancy. Women who are unmarried, who have less than 12 years of education, and who have three or more children continue to have high smoking rates.

The decrease in smoking can be due either to actual changes in smoking behavior or to a shift in the demographic characteristics. The 1984 smoking rates were adjusted to the 1978 rates by the direct adjustment technique. The rates were adjusted for mother's education, age, marital status, and gravidity;

the total rate was also adjusted for race. Seventy-six percent of the 1984 reduction in smoking occurred as a result of changes in smoking behavior rather than in maternal characteristics.

Another perspective of smoking during pregnancy is the level of smoking. Studies show a pattern of decreasing birth weight associated with greater numbers of cigarettes smoked.[1-5] The groups of women with the highest proportion of smokers also tend to be those in which women smoke most heavily, except for whites. Whites have a lower smoking rate but are heavier smokers than nonwhites. The small reduction in heavy smokers has occurred primarily among nonwhites, teen-agers, and women over 30.

The highest smoking rates occur among women who do not have a high-school education, and their smoking rates are not improving. Many of these women are enrolled in public pregnancy- related programs such as Women, Infants and Children (WIC) and Medicaid. Forty-five percent of Missouri WIC mothers smoke during pregnancy, and over a third of all smoking pregnant mothers are enrolled in WIC. These women, who are already receiving regular nutrition and prenatal education from health departments across the country, are a large high-risk captive audience for smoking cessation programs. Moderately successful smoking programs for WIC participants could nearly double the benefit in reduction of low birth weight that the WIC program already provides.[6,7]

In summary, the data from Missouri birth certificates provide unique current and historic information on the smoking patterns of pregnant women. The National Natality Survey and Missouri data agree closely for married women, and the Missouri data permit insights into smoking among unmarried women. The highest smoking rates are found among women who are young, nonwhite, unmarried, not well educated, and who already have children. The overall smoking rates dropped slightly between 1978 and 1984, but an encouraging note is that certain high-risk groups—teenagers and nonwhites—are reducing their level of smoking. The very high smoking rates for women enrolled in public pregnancy-related programs suggests a target for cessation programs.

REFERENCES

1. Schramm WF: Smoking and Pregnancy Outcome. *Mo Med* 1980;77:619-626.
2. Stein Z, Kline J: Smoking, alcohol and reproduction. *Am J Public Health* 1983;73:1154-1156.
3. Niswander JR, Gordon M (eds): *Maternal Characteristics. Section 1. Demographic Characteristics. Cigarette Smoking. In Women and their Pregnancies.* The Collaborative Perinatal Study of the National Institute of Neurological Diseases and Stroke. US Dept Of Health, Education, and Welfare publication No. (NIH) 73-379, 1972, pp 72-80.

4. Kannel WB, Shurtleff D: The Framingham Study: Cigarettes and the development of intermittent claudication. *Geriatrics* 1973;28:61-68.
5. Butler NR, Bonham DG: *Perinatal Mortality*. Edinburgh, E & S Livingston, Ltd, 1963.
6. Stockbauer JW: Evaluation of the Missouri WIC Program: Prenatal Component. Jefferson City, Mo, Dept of Health. *J Am Diet Assoc* 1986:1:61-67.
7. Schramm WF: WIC prenatal participation and its relationship to newborn medicaid costs in Missouri: A cost/benefit analysis. *Am J Public Health* 1985;75:851-857.

23 *Prenatal Smoking and Childhood Morbidity*

Abigail J. Moss, Mary D. Overpeck, Gerry E. Hendershot, Howard J. Hoffman, Heinz W. Berendes

---

Numerous studies since the early 1970s have indicated that maternal smoking has long-lasting adverse effects on a child's health. In 1973, British researchers found significant impairment of physical growth and school-related tasks in the children of mothers who smoked after the fourth month of pregnancy [1] These findings were based on the National Child Development Study, a follow-up study of over 13,000 British children born in 1958 and retested at 7 and 11 years of age. The effect of maternal smoking increased with the number of cigarettes smoked: at 7 and 11 years of age, the children of mothers who smoked ten cigarettes or more a day during pregnancy were, on the average, 1 cm shorter and between 3 and 5 months slower in reading, mathematics, and general ability than children of nonsmoking mothers. Whether these effects are attributable to maternal smoking may not be clear.

Other studies substantiate many of these findings. The California Child Health and Development Study, which followed about 3700 children born at the Oakland Kaiser-Permanente Medical Center between 1959 and 1967, obtained results almost identical to those of the British study.[2] It showed that children of heavy smokers at 5 years of age were almost 1 cm shorter than children of nonsmokers. Similarly, the Canadian study found that 6 1/2-year-old children whose mothers did not smoke during pregnancy had greater mean weights and heights than did children whose mothers smoked.[3]

In a study from Israel, infants of mothers who smoked during pregnancy had significantly more hospital admissions for bronchitis and pneumonia.[4] In addition, a direct relationship was found between hospital admission rates and quantity of cigarettes smoked. Findings similar to these were obtained in a study from northern Finland, in which effects of maternal smoking on morbidity and mortality in children up to the age of 5 years were investigated.[5]

These and other researchers have since found that, even after the data are adjusted for socioeconomic status and other confounding variables, maternal smoking during pregnancy is significantly related to signs of poorer physical, intellectual, and neurologic status in the school-aged child.[6] In 1980, further analysis of data from the British National Child Development Study showed that (1) the mother's smoking during pregnancy was still related to the child's reading and mathematics attainment at age 16, and (2) among boys, there was an association with height, even after adjustment for a number of related background factors.[7]

In another study, published in 1984 by Naeye and Peters, data were used from the Collaborative Perinatal Study of the National Institute of Neurological and Communicative Disorders and Stroke.[8] In this study, siblings were compared whose mothers had smoked in only one of their pregnancies; the siblings were thus genetically and socially similar, which controlled for many parental factors affecting children's mental development. These researchers concluded, "Hyperactivity, short attention span and (slightly) lower scores on spelling and reading tests were more frequent for children whose mothers had smoked throughout pregnancy," although the differences were small.

Not all research studies examining the issue of long-term effects of maternal smoking have produced similar results. Yerushalmy raised the question of whether differences might be due to the characteristics of smokers rather than to smoking.[9] Researchers from John Hopkins University Hospital concluded that, after adjustment for birth weights, children averaged the same weight regardless of mothers' smoking practices during pregnancy, and they differed in height only in the first year. Neurologic status at 1 year and psychological development up to the age of 7 years did not differ significantly between children born to mothers who smoked and those born to mothers who did not. These researchers concluded that "if the child survives the neonatal period, no significant differences beyond the first year are demonstrated in either physical or mental development to seven years of age."[10] These findings have been disputed because of the small sample upon which they were based.[11]

Canadian researchers in another study investigated differences in childrens' neurologic, behavioral, and intellectual development at 7 years of age.[12] After controlling for the many variables affecting a child's development and the different characteristics of smoking and nonsmoking parents, however, the authors were able to find a strong relationship between maternal smoking and intellectual and behavioral development.

In this chapter, the effects of maternal smoking on the postneonatal health of the child are examined through the use of several measures of health status obtained from a population-based survey. These data come from a large, nationally representative sample. This data set differs from the samples used in other studies, which are not representative of the entire at-risk population.

METHODS

The data are derived from the 1981 National Health Interview Survey and this analysis is based on mothers' reports of measures of children's overall health. The health measures used to compare groups of children according to mothers' smoking practices during pregnancy were (1) child's general health, as perceived by the respondent; (2) number of bed days in the past year for health reasons; (3) number of disability days per year; (4) number of chronic conditions and chronic respiratory conditions the child ever had; and (5) number of hospitalizations since birth.

The question used to determine mother's smoking practices during pregnancy was: "During your pregnancy with [child's name], about how many cigarettes a day did you usually smoke?" The questionnaire did not contain a follow-up question, however, to determine whether the mother had quit smoking at any time during the pregnancy. It also did not address the impact of the home and outside environment on the child's health. Specifically, information about the smoking practices of family members at the time of the interview is not known.

RESULTS

Twenty-six percent of mothers reported that they smoked during pregnancy. This estimate is about the same for mothers with children under 3 years of age as for those with 3- to 5-year-olds and is similar to the proportion of married mothers of liveborn infants found in the 1980 National Natality Survey.[13] In this survey, mothers' smoking practices during pregnancy were unknown for about the same proportion of persons with children under 3 and 3 to 5 years (3% compared with 4 1/2%).

Perceived Health Status

Respondents were asked whether they considered the child's overall health to be excellent, good, fair, or poor, compared with other children. Among children under 6 years of age, the proportion reported as being in excellent health decreased significantly if the mother smoked during pregnancy: for nonsmokers, 65% of children were reported as being in excellent health; for women smoking 15 or fewer cigarettes per day, 63% were; and for women smoking 16 or more cigarettes, 52% were.[14]

The differences in the percentage of children considered in excellent health according to the mother's smoking practices during pregnancy only occur for children under 3 years of age, however. Above this age, the proportion of children considered in excellent health is about the same regardless of whether the mother smoked. One out of two children under 3 years of age (51.8%) whose mothers smoked more than 15 cigarettes a day were in excellent health, compared with two out of three children (67%) whose mothers did not smoke ($P < .01$).

Examination of influences of maternal education, parity, age at birth, or the child's race or birth weight on the relationship between maternal smoking and likelihood of excellent health revealed no consistent patterns, apart from the finding that, up to the age of 3 years, children whose mothers did not smoke during pregnancy fared better than did other children.

Days in Bed During the Year

Among all children, the likelihood of spending at least eight days in bed in a year was directly related to the amount the mother smoked during pregnancy: for nonsmoking mothers, 7.4% of children spent at least eight days ill, for light smokers, 10.2%, and for heavy smokers, 12.6%. By age group, however, this trend was significant only for children under 3 years; 7.4% of children for nonsmokers, 11.4% for light smokers, and 16.2% for heavy smokers.

The proportion of children spending 8 or more days in bed differed by race, birth weight, mother's education and age (at the birth), and parity. More young children (proportionately) of mothers who smoked spent at least eight bed days in many of these categories. For example, about twice as many children under 3 years of age who were not first-born and whose mothers smoked stayed in bed eight days or more as did children of similar birth order of nonsmokers (14.5% and 7%)($P < .01$).

Restricted Activity and Bed Disabilities

Differences in the estimates of disability days by age group were only found for children under 3 years of age (Figure 23-1). Children with mothers who smoked during pregnancy had to restrict their activities about five more days a year and stay in bed about seven more days than other children, although only the difference for bed days was significant.

Because the survey's average annual number of restricted activity days and bed days are obtained through questions that use a 2-week recall period, variances are large. Consequently, detecting significant differences between

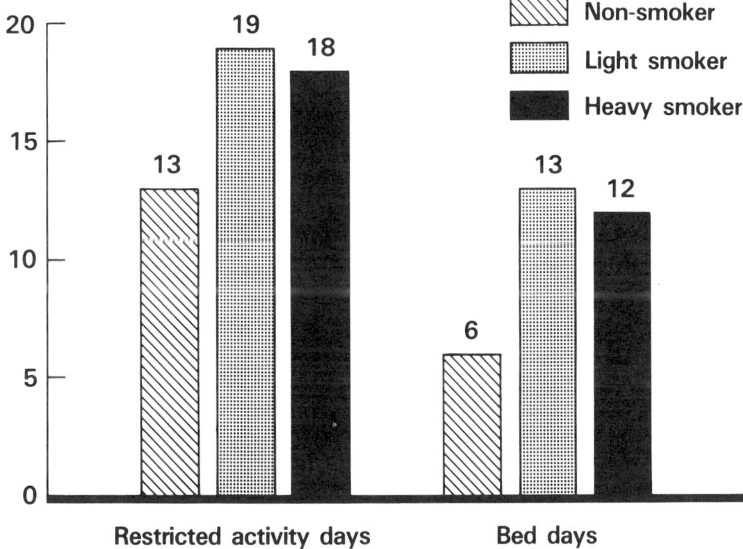

Figure 23-1 Number of restricted activity and bed days per year for children under 3 years (National Health Interview Survey).

estimates that are based on relatively small population groups, such as is the case with these data, only occurs with very large differences.

Number of Chronic Conditions

Mothers were read a list of conditions and asked to indicate which ones their children ever had. The list yielded about 100 chronic ailments of the respiratory, circulatory, digestive, musculoskeletal, skin, sensory, and genitourinary systems.[14] About one of three children under the age of 6 years had had at least one chronic condition. Children under 3 years old whose mothers smoked heavily during pregnancy were significantly more likely to have had at least one chronic condition than were children of nonsmokers (36% compared with 27%). Although the percentage of children under 3 years with one or more chronic conditions is higher for the group whose mothers were heavy smokers than for children of light smokers, the difference is not significant. This pattern was not altered by consideration of maternal age, education, or parity, or of the child's race and birth weight.

Respiratory Conditions

Respiratory conditions were among the most common chronic conditions mentioned; these include asthma, hay fever or allergies, tonsillitis or enlargement of the tonsils or adenoids, tuberculosis and pneumonia, and "any other respiratory, lung, or pulmonary condition." For this last category, conditions were considered chronic only where mothers reported that they had lasted for at least 3 months.

Overall, children of mothers who smoked during pregnancy were more likely to have had chronic asthma, pneumonia, or tonsillitis than other children, although the increase is significant only for asthma. In children under 3 years of age, more than twice as many children whose mothers smoked an average of 16 or more cigarettes daily had respiratory conditions as did children whose mothers did not smoke (15% compared with 6%) ($P < .01$). This contrasts with 3- to-5-year-olds: in this age group the percentages of children with one or more respiratory conditions were about the same, regardless of the mother's smoking practices during pregnancy.

Hospitalizations since Birth

Twenty percent of all children through age 5 years had experienced at least one hospitalization other than birth requiring an overnight or longer stay. A significantly greater proportion of children of smoking mothers than of nonsmokers have been hospitalized (25% compared with 18%) ($P < .01$). Significant differences were also found when a similar comparison was made for children having two or more hospitalizations (8% compared with 4%) ($P < .01$).

Among children under the age of 3 years, children of smokers were significantly more likely to have been hospitalized at least once than children of nonsmokers (20% compared with 12%). Children of heavy smokers were significantly more likely to have been hospitalized at least once than children of light smokers (26% compared with 16%) ($P < .05$). Among 3- to 5-year-olds, the hospitalization likelihood did not differ between the children of heavy and light smokers, but children of mothers who smoked were significantly more likely to have been hospitalized than children of nonsmokers (31% compared with 25%) ($P < .05$).

SUMMARY

All five health status measures analyzed indicate that a mother's smoking during pregnancy impairs a child's health after birth, and the impairment is strongest in children less than 3 years old. These children were perceived to be in poorer health, had more days when poor health interfered with normal activities and resulted in bed rest, and were more likely to have had a chronic condition and to have been hospitalized at least once than children whose mothers did not smoke. Among these children, a direct relationship exists between the number of cigarettes smoked and the health impairment of the child. These patterns generally hold even when maternal age and parity at birth, education, and the child's birth weight and age are considered.

The effects that maternal smoking has on children's health appear to diminish with time. Except for hospitalizations, the estimates for all health indicators were similar for 3- to 5-year-old children of smoking and nonsmoking mothers. Similarly, no significant differences were found for this age group in the health status estimates between children whose mothers were light or heavy smokers.

These findings are consistent with those from other studies and clearly provide further evidence that smoking in pregnancy adversely affects later health of young children.

REFERENCES

1. Butler NR, Goldstein H: Smoking in pregnancy and subsequent child development. *Br Med J* 1973;4:573-575.
2. Wingerd J, Schoen EJ: Factors influencing length at birth and height at five years. *Pediatrics* 1974;53:737-741.
3. Dunn HG, McBurney A, Ingram S, et al: Maternal cigarette smoking during pregnancy and the child's subsequent development: I. Physical growth to the age of 6 1/2 years. *Can J Public Health* 1976;67:499-505.
4. Harlap S, Davies AM: Infant admissions to hospital and maternal smoking. *Lancet* 1974;1:529-532.
5. Rantakallio P: Relationship of maternal smoking to morbidity and mortality of the child up to the age of five. *Acta Paediatr Scand* 1978;67:621-631.
6. Rantakallio P: A follow-up study to the age of 14 of children whose mothers smoked during pregnancy. *Acta Paediatr Scand* 1983;72:747-753.
7. Fogelman K: Smoking in pregnancy and subsequent development of the child. *Child Care Health and Dev* 1980;6:233-251.
8. Naeye RL, Peters EC: Mental development of children whose mothers smoked during pregnancy. *Obstet Gynecol* 1984;64:601-607.
9. Yerushalmy J: The relationship of parents' cigarette smoking to outcome of pregnancy—implications as to the problem of inferring causation from observed associations. *Am J Epidemiol* 1971;93:433-456.
10. Hardy JB, Mellits ED: Does maternal smoking during pregnancy have a long-term effect on the child? *Lancet* 1972;2:1332-1336.
11. Donovan JW: Effects of child on maternal smoking during pregnancy. *Lancet* 1973;1:376.
12. Dunn HG, McBurney A, Ingram S, et al: Maternal cigarette smoking during pregnancy and the child's subsequent develop- ment: II. Neurological and intellectual maturation to the age of 6 1/2 years. *Can J Public Health* 1977;64:43-50.
13. National Center for Health Statistics: *Maternal smoking and drinking behavior before and during pregnancy: Health United States, 1983.* Hyattsville, Md, National Center for Health Statistics. US Dept of Health and Human Services publication No. (PHS)84-1232, 45, 1983.
14. National Center for Health Statistics: *Current Estimates from the National Health Interview Survey, United States, 1981.* Hyattsville, Md, National Center for Health Statistics, Vital and Health Statistics Series 10: Data from the National Health Survey, No. 141. US Dept of Health and Human Services publication No. (PHS)83-1569,93, 1983.

24 *Sharing the Cigarette: The Effects of Smoking in Pregnancy*

Benjamin P. Sachs

The fetus is potentially exposed to many drugs and environmental toxins. The thalidomide disaster focused the attention of the public and the medical profession on the serious consequences of some of these exposures. Although the hazards of smoking in pregnancy are not as dramatic as the teratogenic effects of thalidomide, the consequences are nevertheless profound. Physicians are well aware of the risks to adults posed by smoking but often fail to emphasize similar education and prevention efforts for the mother-to-be. Gynecologists have a unique opportunity in their role as primary care physicians for many young women. This chapter reviews the pathophysiology and epidemiology of smoking in pregnancy.

Women may smoke or be exposed to cigarette smoke in the home, the workplace, and in public places. The main risk for the involuntary smoker is carbon monoxide, as nicotine quickly settles out of the air.[1] The amount of carbon monoxide exposure depends on the number and type of cigarettes smoked, the ventilation of the enclosed space, and the size of the area. The maximum permissible exposure level is nine parts of carbon monoxide per million of air.[2] As these safety guidelines can be exceeded in many situations, a mother and fetus are clearly at risk.

FETAL PHYSIOLOGY

Understanding the physiologic accommodation of the fetus to life in utero is important to comprehend the effects of smoking. The fetus normally resides in a state of "physiologic hypoxia," with a mean umbilical vein P_{O_2} of 35 torr and a mean umbilical artery P_{O_2} of 22 torr (as measured on sheep breathing air at sea level).[3] The low oxygen tension maintains the patency of the ductus arteriosus and the constriction of the pulmonary vasculature in utero. The fetus lives in this state of physiologic hypoxia through a number of mechanisms: (1) fetal hemoglobin (HbF), which has greater oxygen affinity than adult hemoglobin (HbA); (2) high hematocrit; and (3) high cardiac output due to faster heart rate and higher stroke volume. All these physiologic mechanisms allow the fetus to survive at this low P_{O_2}, but also render it susceptible to tobacco smoke.

Aerobic metabolism depends on an efficient mechanism for the transport of oxygen from the atmosphere to the tissues. Because of the low solubility of O_2 in plasma, an efficient O_2 carrier is required. In adult humans this is Hb A, and in the fetus for most of gestation it is principally Hb F. These hemoglobins differ in their O_2 affinity at different partial pressures of oxygen. Compared with the oxyhemoglobin dissociation curve for adult hemoglobin, the fetal hemoglobin curve is shifted to the left, with a lower P_{50} (Figure 24-1). These curves can be shifted by changes in P_{CO_2},[4] pH,[4] temperature,[5] and 2,3-diphosphoglycerate (2,3-DPG).[6,7] In 1967, Benesch and Benesch[6] and Chanutin and Curnish[7] independently demonstrated that an increase in 2,3-DPG results in decreased HbO_2 affinity (a shift in the HbO_2 dissociation curve to the right).[6,7] This organic phosphate, which is the principal end metabolite of glucose in the red blood cell, plays a major role in the regulation of O_2 transport.[8] However, 2,3-DPG in the fetus has only 40% of the effect on HbO_2 affinity, as a result of an amino acid substitution.[9] In

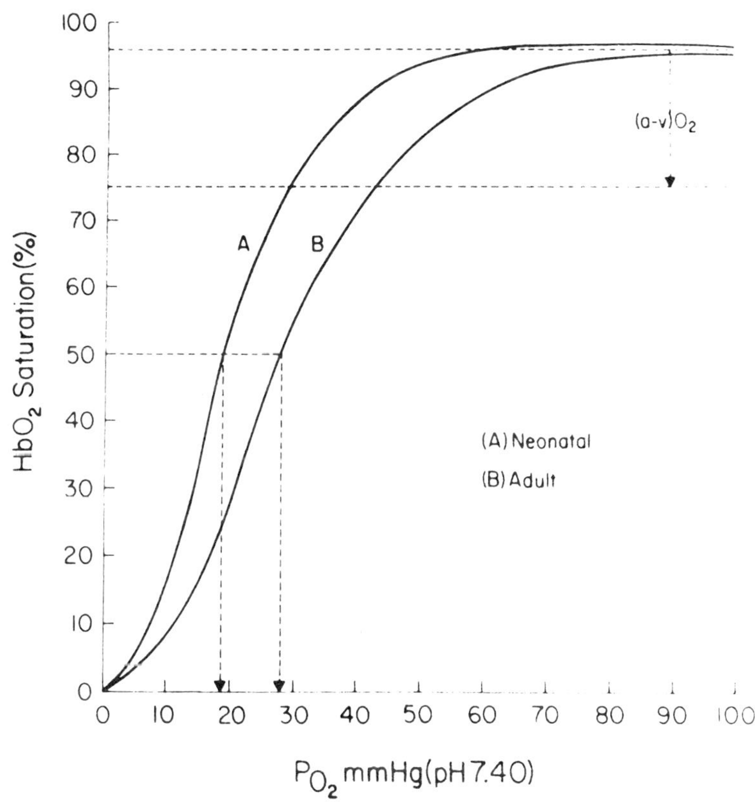

Figure 24-1 Oxyhemoglobin dissociation curve. A=Hb F, P50=19 torr. B=Hb A, P50=27 torr.

response to acute or chronic hypoxia, there is an elevation in 2,3-DPG and a decrease in HbO_2 affinity.[10,11] These changes maintain the end capillary PO_2 with the least demand on cardiac output.[12]

FETAL RESPONSE TO CARBON MONOXIDE

Carbon monoxide from cigarette smoke not only causes fetal hypoxia, but also prevents an adequate physiologic response to this insult. The affinity for hemoglobin of carbon monoxide is 200 times that of oxygen.[13,14] Furthermore, Hb F has a higher affinity for carbon monoxide than Hb A. When Hb F combines with carbon monoxide, there is a left shift in the O_2 dissociation curve. These changes lead to a decrease in the oxygen-carrying capacity of the blood and a decrease in the offloading of oxygen at the tissue level, resulting in a functional anemia. After five to six hours, carbon monoxide levels in the fetus are in equilibrium with maternal levels.[15] Carbon monoxide lasts longer in the fetus, which is less able to metabolize it.[2] Just two packs of cigarettes per day smoked by the mother results in a 10% concentration of carboxyhem-oglobin, which is equivalent to a 60% reduction in blood flow to the fetus.[2,15] As the fetus is normally in a low oxygen environment, there is little margin for safety with respect to tissue oxygenation. Furthermore, the fetus is unable to compensate by increasing cardiac output, as its cardiac output is already at or near peak.[2] Thus, the fetus is unable to compensate adequately for carbon monoxide from cigarette smoke.[2,16]

These findings were also seen in a study of the effect of smoking on 100 mother-infant pairs, equally divided between smoking and nonsmoking mothers.[17] The smokers had no significant change in the levels of 2,3-DPG and the P_{50} values, but their hematocrits were increased by a small but significant amount. There was a significant difference for the smoke-exposed infants in their Hb F and P_{50} values, but no change in the 2,3-DPG levels. These changes reflect an inefficient compensatory mechanism and emphasize the sensitivity of the fetus to an increased concentration of carbon monoxide from cigarettes. In the sensitivity of its response, the fetus can be compared to the canaries that used to be taken underground by miners to detect carbon monoxide.

CONSTITUENTS OF TOBACCO SMOKE

Burning the tobacco leaf results in gases and tiny droplets of tar. The principal gaseous ingredients are nicotine, carbon monoxide, and cyanide; in addition there are numerous cancer-producing substances.[18] Carbon monoxide is a principal constituent of tobacco smoke.

One puff of a cigarette is equivalent to an intravenous injection of 0.1 mg of nicotine (2 mg of nicotine per cigarette).[17,19] Nicotine acts on the adrenal glands and causes an increase in norepinephrine, epinephrine, and acetylcholine.[20,21] It leads to decreased uteroplacental perfusion and, furthermore, crosses the placenta to affect the fetal cardiovascular system. It has been shown to cause a rise in the blood pressure and respiratory rate of the fetus and affects the gastrointestinal, genitourinary, and central nervous system. Nicotine causes addiction, or so-called habituating behavior.[17,19,22]

PLACENTAL MORPHOLOGY

Knowledge of placental changes is important to understanding the effect of smoking on the fetus. Van der Veen and Fox examined by light and electron microscopy 100 placentas, 72 from smokers and the rest from nonsmokers.[23] They found a relative hypertrophy of the placentas from smokers, which was thought to be a response to chronic hypoxia. In addition, they found a number of changes consistent with chronic ischemia: (*a*) a decrease in the vasculosyncytial membrane, (*b*) a decrease in cytotrophoblastic cell proliferation, (*c*) decreased pinocytosis and trophoblastic secretor activity, and (*d*) focal syncytial necrosis. These morphologic changes in the placenta, which are seen in chronic ischemia, are consistent with our understanding of the effects of carbon monoxide and nicotine on the fetus.

THE EFFECT OF SMOKING ON BIRTH WEIGHT

In 1953 Simpson began her study of the effect of smoking on pregnancy. Her 1957 report[24] showed that, in a population of 7499 women in San Bernardino County, California, there was a near doubling of the prematurity rate among smokers and that the rate of premature births correlated with the number of cigarettes smoked. Since this report, there have been many others on this subject, not all supporting her findings. To understand the controversial areas, three important issues will be addressed here. First, is smoking causative of or associated with low birth weight (LBW)? Second, is the LBW due to intrauterine growth retardation and/or prematurity? Third, what is the mechanism for the observed changes?

There have been many studies of the effect of smoking on LBW.[25-35] Some showed an increased incidence of small-for-gestational-age infants (SGA)[25-28,34,35] and decreased birth length,[26-29] and others showed a higher incidence of premature infants appropriate for gestational age (AGA).[25-28]

Yerushalmy[31] in 1971 argued that the lower birth weight was caused by characteristics of the smoker as well as by smoking itself. Since the reduction in birth weight was seen in mothers who first began smoking after their pregnancy, he was pointing out the problem of inferring causation from observed associations. Clearly, many potential confounding variables can affect birth weight, including maternal age, race, sex, and maternal weight gain. Yerushalmy and others[31-34] have argued that the poor maternal weight gain in pregnancy commonly seen among smokers accounts for the lower birth weight. In a 1978 report supported by the Council for Tobacco Research,[34] this argument was made without substantiating evidence. Furthermore, this paper claimed that there was a possibility that nicotine could induce a physiologic response "serving to alleviate bioenergetic deficiency in some individuals." In this view both smoking and low birth weight are "symptoms of deficient maternal bioenergetic systems." The author even claimed that for some patients nicotine from cigarette smoke may be beneficial for the mother and the fetus.

These reports are in the minority in maintaining that there is no link between cigarette smoking and low birth weight. The data at the very least demonstrate a strong association, if not actual causation.[25-28] The 1983 report of the Surgeon General[25] on the consequences of smoking in women reviewed five studies with respect to the issue of low birth weight. These studies comprise nearly 113,000 births in the United States, Canada, and Wales. It was found that between 21% and 39% of the incidence of low birth weight could be attributed to maternal cigarette smoking.

In a study[36] addressing this issue, which was conducted on 8000 pregnancies, the effect on birth weight was found to be independent of dietary intake or nutritional status and was present regardless of prepregnancy weight or weight gain. Furthermore, a dose response was seen: the more cigarettes smoked, the lower the birth weight. Genetic factors were ruled out by studying information obtained from two successive pregnancies, in only one of which the mother smoked. In these cases, there was a clear link between smoking and low birth weight. Furthermore, the analysis showed the effect on birth weight was independent of socioeconomic class, maternal age, or birth order.

There are two good arguments to counter those who believe that smoking mothers eat less and therefore have smaller babies. First, one would expect to find poor maternal weight gain if the fetus is growth-retarded, as 30% to 40% of the weight gain in the last trimester is due to fetal growth. Hence, the observation of low maternal weight gain and SGA infants. Second, there is no clear connection between poor maternal nutrition and the incidence of SGA infants.[37] Even in studies conducted in as extreme a situation as the Second World War, the mother had to be severely malnourished for there to be any effect on birth weight. Moreover, these results were confounded by poor prenatal care at that time.[38,39]

A recent randomized clinical trial[40] of changes in maternal smoking and its effect on birth weight has lent support to a relationship between smoking and birth weight. Nine hundred thirty-five pregnant mothers were randomly assigned to treatment and control groups. The former achieved a 43% reduction in smoking, while 20% of the control group stopped. Salivary thiocyanate levels were measured in both groups to quantify the cigarette exposure. The authors reported for singleton liveborn infants that the treatment group had a mean birth weight 92 g heavier and mean birth length 0.6 cm longer than the control group infants. These findings were independent of gestational age. This small weight gain seen among the treatment group was the average for the whole group and included 67% of mothers who continued to smoke, although less frequently.

The only other experimental study was that of Donovan,[41] which did not show an effect. However, Donovan was unable to quantify the amount of smoking with salivary thiocyanate levels. A question that needs further research is: What is the effect of stopping smoking in pregnancy? Is this situation analogous to that of the opiate addict, in which we know that withdrawal of the drug can adversely affect the fetus?

Some studies have reported an increase in the incidence of premature deliveries[42-44] associated with maternal smoking. However, many of these studies were based on data from birth records, which are notoriously poor in the assessment of gestational age. The birth weight differential between infants born to smokers and nonsmokers is between 150 and 300 g.[25] Vital records data are not sensitive enough to detect these changes in gestational age. The magnitude of the effect of smoking on the incidence of prematurity is unknown. There is a strong association between cigarette smoking and abruptio placentae[25,27,30] and premature rupture of membranes,[25,35] both being clinical conditions that can lead to premature birth. One hypothesis for this association is nicotine; its pharmacologic effects on the placental vasculature have been discussed.

The mechanisms whereby smoking affects fetal growth are controversial. Some of the suggestions have included hypoxia, vascular problems, maternal nutrition, and a direct fetal effect. Chronic fetal hypoxia and impaired fetal circulation go hand in hand. We have seen that carbon monoxide has a toxic effect to which the fetus is poorly able to respond because of thephysiologic hypoxia in utero and the fact that fetal cardiac function is near maximum.[2,16] The pathologic role of nicotine has been well described.[20,21,44-47] Nicotine can cause vasoconstriction, which causes release of acetylcholine, epinephrine, and norepinephrine.[20,21] Some studies have reported a decrease in venous blood flow due to smoking or chewing tobacco.[45,48] However, not all agree with these findings.[34] Two other mechanisms that may compound the effects of carbon monoxide and nicotine are (1) an inhibition of carbonic-anhydrase, which can lead to tissue hypoxia, and (2) the hydrocyanic acid present in tobacco smoke in its conversion to thiocyanate, which may cause tissue hypoxia.

SUMMARY OF THE EFFECT OF SMOKING ON BIRTH WEIGHT

The preponderance of evidence points to a very strong association, if not a cause-and-effect relationship, between smoking and intrauterine growth retardation. The average deficit in full term infants born to smokers is 300 g.

Furthermore, there is a clear dose response between the number of cigarettes smoked and the weight of the newborn. The epidemiologic evidence is supported by our understanding of the effects of carbon monoxide and nicotine on the fetus. We have reviewed the pharmacologic effects of these drugs, and it is clear that the fetus is poorly able to respond to these insults. In addition, the placental changes described support the concept of chronic hypoxia in utero due to cigarette smoke. There is also an increased incidence of premature infants, which may in addition be small for gestational age. A possible mechanism for this prematurity is through the effects of nicotine and the relationship to abruptio placentae. The pathophysiology of premature labor is not understood. We recognize pathologic conditions associated with prematurity, such as chorioamnionitis and pregnancy-induced hypertension. The clear association between cigarette smoking and prematurity must be recognized, even though its mechanism is not understood. Most evidence points to an effect of smoking rather than of the smoker. The effect is still seen after the data are adjusted for confounding factors such as maternal age, race, socioeconomic status, and sex of the infant. Because an unrecognized potential confounding factor may have accounted for the findings in the retrospective studies, Sexton and Hebel[40] undertook a randomized clinical trial. This study clearly supports a cause-and-effect relationship.

For many studies, it is unclear whether the effect of smoking is on fetal growth or prematurity. A 300-g deficit in a full-term infant weighing more than 2500 g is not as relevant clinically as it would be in the low birth weight SGA and AGA infant. It is therefore important to make this distinction in educating gynecologists and other health care providers.

OTHER EFFECTS OF SMOKING AND PREGNANCY

Perinatal Mortality

Maternal smoking is strongly associated with an estimated 4600 infant deaths in the United States each year.[25] A number of studies have shown an increase in the incidence of stillbirths and neonatal and postneonatal deaths.[24,25,35,49-51] Some of these reports showed that the increase in perinatal mortality was independent of decreased birth weight.[25,27,35] However, a few studies[52-54] have shown no increase in the incidence in perinatal mortality. Some of the controversy may be explained by a point made by Goldstein,[55] that the sample size required to examine the effect of smoking in the perinatal mortality would have to exceed 10,000 women and that the effect on the perinatal mortality rate is likely to be very small, especially for babies weighing over 3000 g. The randomized clinical study by Sexton and Hebel[40] showed no difference in the incidence of perinatal mortality, although this study was never designed to show a difference and had less than sufficient sample sizes. Of interest is a study by Meyer and Tonascia[35] analyzing data from the Ontario Perinatal Mortality Study, which showed a 20% increased risk of a perinatal death for women who smoked less than a pack a day and a 35% increase for those who smoked more than a pack a day. The deaths were associated with a high incidence of bleeding during pregnancy due to abruptio placentae, placenta previa, and premature rupture of the membranes.

Low Apgar Scores

Garn et al,[56] using data from the Collaborative Perinatal Project on the one- and five-minute Apgar scores of 43,492 infants, showed that there was a fourfold increased incidence of low Apgar scores if the mother smoked more than two packs of cigarettes a day. These findings were independent of race or gestational age of the baby. They also showed that the babies exposed to cigarette smoke had higher hematocrits and cord carbon monoxide levels.

Abruptio Placentae and Other Antepartum Hemorrhages

A number of studies[25,27,35] have shown an increased incidence of abruptio placentae among smoking mothers. Others have reported an increase in the incidence of placenta previa.[25,35] It is hard to understand the cause-and-effect relationship between cigarette smoking and abnormal placement of the placenta. Many of these studies were conducted before the era of modern ultrasonography, which has enabled us to localize the placenta accurately, and so there may have been diagnostic errors.

Premature Rupture of Membranes

A few studies have reported an increased incidence of premature rupture of membranes.[25,35,57] The mechanism is unknown, and it is unclear whether there is cause and effect or an association.

Respiratory Distress Syndrome (RDS)

In their study of the efficacy of steroids for preventing RDS, the Collaborative Group on Antenatal Steroid Therapy found a lower incidence of RDS in babies exposed to cigarette smoke in utero.[58] The findings were significant after the data were adjusted for treatment and risk factors. The relationship is not surprising, as the incidence of RDS is known to be lower in "stressed" or SGA infants.

Pregnancy-Induced Hypertension

Pregnant women who smoke have been reported to have a lower incidence of hypertensive disorders.[25,35], The mechanism is not understood.

Birth Defects

In a study of 67,609 singleton pregnancies in Cardiff, Wales,[59] between 1965 and 1976, the overall incidence of congenital anomalies was 2.8% for both smokers and nonsmokers. There was no dose-response effect for malformations except for neural-tube defects, which were increased in infants of heavy smokers. However, the potential confounding variable in this study was socioeconomic status, which appeared to be a stronger correlate than smoking per se. In a case-controlled study from Sweden,[60] in which 66 infants with cleft lip and/or cleft palate, 66 with closure defects, and 261 controls were examined, significantly more women having infants with cleft lip or cleft palate smoked compared with controls. The findings were independent of other drug use. Hemminki et al[61] studied 3300 children with defects between 1967 and 1977 in the Finnish Register of Congenital Malformations. They carried out a multivariate analysis of this retrospective data set and found that, when controlling for 13 possible confounding variables, smoking was not a teratogen. In summary, most of the large controlled studies have been unable to show a teratogenic effect of cigarette smoking.

Long-Term Morbidity

There appears to be a long-term effect of cigarette smoking on surviving children.[25,62-64] However, the effect on child development cannot be completely separated from such potential confounding variables as socioeconomic status, education, and passive smoking. In a study of over 5000 children in the British National Child Development Study, Davie et al[63] and Goldstein[64] used a multifactorial analysis to show reduced reading attainment at 7 years of age, in children whose mothers had smoked more than ten cigarettes a day; there were retardations of 3 months in general ability, 4 months in reading skills, and 5 months in mathematics. However, none of these findings was statistically significant.

IS THERE LONG-TERM RISK OF CANCER FOLLOWING IN UTERO EXPOSURE TO CIGARETTES?

Everson,[65] in a recent article, proposed an association between cigarette smoking and long-term risk of cancer to the infant. His argument was based on clinical observations and animal experimentation. It was first reported in the 1940s that urethane was a transplacental carcinogen in mice.[66,67] Since this early report, more than 30 agents have been identified as active transplacental carcinogens. The best known transplacental carcinogen is diethylstilbestrol (DES), which has been associated with vaginal clear cell adenocarcinoma in women whose mothers received DES in pregnancy.[68,69] Furthermore, hydantoin, used to treat epilepsy, has been associated with neuroblastomas and a malignant mesenchymoma.[70]

A number of agents that are potent transplacental carcinogens in animals can be found in cigarette smoke. These are benzopyrene, urethane, nitrosamines, and hydrazines.[71-72] However, there is only indirect evidence for their ability to cross the placenta in humans. The rapid growth of the fetus in utero is thought to make it more susceptible to transplacental carcinogens. There is some experimental evidence in animals to support this hypothesis.[73,74] In addition, the carcinogens may increase sensitivity to later exposure to carcinogens.[72,75] Epidemiological studies in humans have not been conclusive. Neutal and Buck,[76] for a cohort of 89,302 infants in 1971, reported a relative risk of 1.3 (95% confidence limits 0.8 - 2.2) for cancer among offspring of women who smoke during pregnancy. Most of the other studies examining this issue had too few numbers to study what is probably a low-incidence problem.[77,78]

FETAL TOBACCO SYNDROME

It has been recommended that the findings discussed above be described as "fetal tobacco syndrome."[79] The introduction of the term "fetal alcohol syndrome" clearly increased the consciousness level of the public and the medical profession as to the hazards of drinking in pregnancy. Through the introduction of the term fetal tobacco syndrome, there are potentially a number of benefits: (1) uniform diagnostic criteria, (2) heightened awareness by the public and medical profession, (3) more precise epidemiologic assessment of populations at risk, and (4) more careful evaluation of smoking intervention programs. The criteria proposed by the Centers for Disease Control are:

1. Mother smoked five or more cigarettes a day throughout the pregnancy.

2. Mother had no evidence of hypertension during pregnancy, especially (*a*) no preeclampsia and (*b*) documentation of normal blood pressure at least once after the first trimester.

3. The newborn has symmetrical growth retardation (greater than 37 weeks), defined as (*a*) birth weight less than 2500 g and (*b*) a ponderal index (weight in grams/length in centimeters)[1] greater than 2.32.

4. There is no other obvious cause of intrauterine growth retardation (eg, congenital infection or anomaly).

CONCLUSION

There is overwhelming evidence that smoking is harmful to the fetus. The epidemiologic data that examines the relationship between smoking and fetal effects can be summarized as follows:

1. A decrease in birth weight in term infants of between 150 and 300 g: Most studies have shown that this is an effect of smoking and not of the smoker. For LBW infants (less than 2500 g) in the United States, Canada, and Wales, 21% to 39% of the cases could be attributed to maternal smoking.

2. Increased incidence of prematurity[25-28]: The risk of a preterm birth in these studies was 36% to 47% higher than in•controls and of all the preterm births 11% to 14% were attributable to smoking. In many of the studies it is unclear whether the effect of smoking is on fetal growth or prematurity. A 300-g deficit in a full-term infant weighing more than 2500 g is not as relevant clinically as it would be in a low birth weight SGA or AGA infant. It is therefore important to make this distinction in educating gynecologists and other health care providers.

3. There is a clear dose-response effect on birth weight, with light smokers having a 54% and heavy smokers a 130% increase in the frequency of infants weighing less than 2500 g at birth.

4. Increased perinatal mortality: An estimated 4600 infants die each year in the United States as a result of maternal smoking.[25,26,35,49-51]

5. Increased incidence of low Apgar scores: There is a reported fourfold increase in the incidence of depressed newborn infants among mothers who smoked two or more packs per day.[56]

6. Increased incidence of abruptio placentae.[25,27,35]

7. Increased incidence of premature rupture of membranes.[25,35,57]

8. Decreased incidence of respiratory distress syndrome.[58]

9. Decreased incidence of pregnancy-induced hypertension.[25,35]

10. Birth defects: Most studies have shown no teratogenic effect of cigarette smoking.[59-61]

11. Increased incidence of long-term morbidity in infants exposed to cigarette smoke in utero. However, in most of these studies it is difficult to control for potential confounding variables, such as socioeconomic status and the effect of passive smoking.[25,62-64]

12. Question of increased long-term cancer risk to the infant exposed in utero: At this stage, this is still a hypothesis, but it is supported by a large body of experimental data in animals. However, in human epidemiologic studies, it may be hard to control for potential confounding variables, and the sample sizes would have to be very large.[65-70] The epidemiologic evidence is supported by our understanding of the physiology of fetal oxygenation and the response of the fetus to carbon monoxide. Furthermore, nicotine and other substances clearly affect fetal oxygenation. The observed placental changes further support these mechanisms.

The effect of passive smoking on the pregnant woman has not received sufficient attention. If a pregnant woman who does not smoke is exposed to smoke, the effect could conceivably be as important as if she smoked herself. More research is required in this area, but this should not delay public health programs in addressing this issue.

A number of areas require further research, including clearer elucidation of the mechanism and the magnitude of the effect of maternal smoking on prematurity. These areas encompass the extent of the long-term neurologic impairment and cancer risk for infants exposed in utero to cigarette smoke and the effect of passive smoking on the fetus.

Because the case that smoking affects the fetus is so strong, it is clear that obstetricians, as primary care providers for women, and other health professionals who come into contact with pregnant women have an obligation help women to stop smoking. There are admittedly important areas that require further research. However, there is without doubt sufficient evidence at this stage to warrant a large public health campaign.

REFERENCES

1. US Dept of Health, Education and Welfare: Involuntary smoking, in *Health Consequences of Smoking*. Government Printing Office, 1975.
2. Longo LD: The biological effects of carbon monoxide on the pregnant woman, fetus and newborn infant. *Am J Obstet Gynecol* 1977;129:69-103.
3. Meschia G: Placental respiratory gas exchange and fetal oxygenation, in Creasy R, Resnick R (eds): *Maternal and Fetal Medicine Principles and Practice*. Philadelphia, WB Saunders Co 1984, pp 274-285.
4. Bohr C, Hasselbalch KA, Krough A: Ueber einer in biologischer Beziehung wichtigen Einfluss, den die Kohlensäurespannung des Blutes auf der Sauerstoffbindung übt. *Scand Arch Physiol* 1904;16:402-412.
5. Barcroft J, King WOR: The effect of temperature on the dissociation curve of blood. *J Physiol* 1909;39:374-384.
6. Benesch R, Benesch RE: The effect of organic phosphates from the human erythrocyte on the allosteric properties of hemoglobin. *Biochem Biophys Res Commun* 1967;26:162-167.
7. Chanutin A, Curnish RR: Effect of organic phosphates on the oxygen equilibrium of human erythrocytes. *Arch Biochem Biophys* 1967;121:96-102.
8. Rapaport S, Nieradt C: In wieweit verläuft die Glykolyse im saugetiererythrozyten über 2,3-Diphosphoglycerinsaure: Über eine Variant der glykolyischer Zyclus auf dem Niveau der Phosphoglycerensaueren. *Biochem Ztschr* 1955;326:231-236.
9. Orzalasi MM, Hay WW: Regulation of oxygen affinity of fetal blood. I. In vitro experiments and results in normal infants. *Pediatrics* 1971;48:857-864.
10. Oski FA, Gottlieb AJ, Delivoria-Papadopoulos M, et al: Red cell 2,3-diphosphoglycerate levels in subjects with chronic hypoxemia. *N Engl J Med* 1967;280:1165-1166.
11. Lenfant C, Warp P, Aucutt C, et al: Effect of chronic hypoxia on the O_2-

Hb dissociation curve and respiratory gas transport in man. *Respir Physiol* 1969;7:7-30.
12. Rossoff L, Zelden R, Hew E, et al: Changes in blood P50: effects on oxygen delivery when arterial hypoxemia is due to shunting. *Chest* 1980;77:142-146.
13. Rand PW, Norton JM, Barker ND, et al: Responses to graded hypoxia at high and low 2,3-diphosphoglycerate concentrations. *J Appl Physiol* 1973;34:827-832.
14. Longo LD: Carbon monoxide effects on oxygenization of the fetus in utero. *Science* 1976;194:523-525.
15. Longo LD, Hill EP: Carbon monoxide uptake and elimination in fetal and maternal sheep. *Am J Physiol* 1977;232:324.
16. Bureau MA, Shapcott D, Berthiaume Y: Maternal cigarette smoking and fetal oxygen transport; a study of P50, 2,3-diphosphoglycerate, total hemoglobin, hematocrit, and type F hemoglobin in fetal blood. *Pediatrics* 1983;72:22-26.
17. Royal College of Physicians of London: The chemistry and pharmacology of tobacco smoke, in *Smoking and Health Now*, London, Pitman Medical, 1971, pp 35-47.
18. Fried PA, Oxorn H: *Smoking For Two: Cigarettes and Pregnancy*. New York, The Free Press, 1980.
19. US Dept of Health, Education, and Welfare: Harmful constituents, in *The Health Consequences of Smoking: A Report of the Surgeon General.* Government Printing Office, 1978, pp 229-235.
20. Monheit AG, van Vunakis H, Key TC, et al: Maternal and fetal cardiovascular effects of nicotine infusion in pregnant sheep. *Am J Obstet Gynecol* 1983;145:290-296.
21. Manning FA, Walker D, Feyerabend C: The effect of nicotine on fetal breathing movements in conscious pregnant ewes. *Obstet Gynecol* 1978;52:563-568.
22. Royal College of Physicians of London: *Smoking or Health. The Third Report of the Royal College of Physicians of London.* London, Pitman Medical, 1977, p 128.
23. Van der Veen F, Fox H: The effects of cigarette smoking on the human placenta: a light and electron microscopic study. *Placenta* 1982;3:243-248.
24. Simpson WJ: A preliminary report on cigarette smoking and the incidence of prematurity. *Am J Obstet Gynecol* 1957;73:808-814.
25. US Dept of Health and Human Services: *The Health Consequences of Smoking for Women: A Report of the Surgeon General*, US Dept of Health and Human Services publication No 410-889/1284, 1983, pp 191-249.
26. Naeye RL: Effects of maternal cigarette smoking on the fetus and placenta. *Br J Obstet Gynecol* 1978;85:732-737.
27. US Dept of Health, Education, and Welfare: Pregnancy and infant health, in *Smoking and Health.* Government Printing Office 1979, pp 8-1 - 8-93.
28. Stein ZA, Susser M: Intrauterine growth retardation: Epidemiological issues and public health significance. *Semin Perinatol* 1984;8:5-15.
29. Miller HC, Hasseinein K, Hensleigh PA: Fetal growth retardation in relation to maternal smoking and weight gain in pregnancy. *Am J Obstet Gynecol* 1976;125:55-60.
30. Smoking and Intrauterine Growth Retardation, editorial. *Lancet* 1979;1:536-537.

31. Yerushalmy J: The relationship of parents' cigarette smoking to outcome of pregnancy: Implications as to the problem of inferring causation from observed associations. *Am J Epidemiol* 1971;93:443-446.
32. Yerushalmy J: Mother's cigarette smoking and survival of infant. *Am J Obstet Gynecol* 1964;88:505-518.
33. Yerushalmy J: Infants with low birth weight born before their mothers started to smoke cigarettes. *Am J Obstet Gynecol* 1972;112:277-284.
34. Hickey RJ, Clelland RC, Bowers EJ: Maternal smoking, birth weight, infant death, and the self-selection problem. *Am J Obstet Gynecol* 1978;131:805-811.
35. Meyer NB, Tonascia JA: Maternal smoking, pregnancy complications and perinatal mortality. *Am J Obstet Gynecol* 1977;128:494-592.
36. Naeye RL: Influence of maternal cigarette smoking during pregnancy on fetal and childhood growth. *Obstet Gynecol* 1981;57:18-21.
37. Stein Z, Susser M, Rush D: Prenatal nutrition and birth weight: Experiments and quasi experiments in the past decade. *J Reprod Med* 1978;21:287-299.
38. Antonov AW: Children born during the seige of Leningrad in 1942. *J Pediatr* 1947;30:250-256.
39. Smith CA: Effects of maternal undernutrition upon the newborn infant in Holland. *J Pediatr* 1947;30:299-303.
40. Sexton M, Hebel JR: A clinical trial of change in maternal smoking and its effect on birthweight. *JAMA* 1984;251:911-915.
41. Donovan JW: Randomized controlled trial of anti-smoking advice in pregnancy. *Br J Prev Soc Med* 1977;31:6-12.
42. Buncher CR: Cigarette smoking and duration of pregnancy. *Am J Obstet Gynecol* 1969;103:942-946.
43. Lowe CR: Effect of mothers' smoking habits on birth weight of their children. *Br Med J* 1959;2:673-675.
44. Yerushalmy J: The relationship of parents' cigarette smoking to outcome of pregnancy—implications as to the problem of inferring causation from observed associations. *Am J Epidemiol* 1971;9:443-456.
45. Lehtovirta P, Forss M: The acute effect of smoking on intervillous blood flow of the placenta. *Br J Obstet Gynecol* 1978;85:729-731.
46. Lehtovirta P, Forss M, Kariniemi V, et al: Acute effects of smoking on fetal heart-rate variability. *Br J Obstet Gynaecol* 1983;90:3-6.
47. Lehtovirta P, Forss M, Rauramo I, et al: Acute effects of nicotine on fetal heart rate variability. *Br J Obstet Gynaecol* 1983;90:710-715.
48. Verma RC, Chansoriya M, Kaul KK: Effect of tobacco chewing by mothers on fetal outcome. *Indian Pediatr* 1983;20:105-111.
49. Butler NR, Bonham DG: *Perinatal Mortality. The First Report of the 1958 British Perinatal Mortality Survey.* Edinburgh, E & S Livingstone, Ltd, 1963.
50. Comstock GW, Lundin FE Jr: Parental smoking and perinatal mortality. *Am J Obstet Gynecol* 1967;98:708-712.
51. Ravenholt RT, Levinski MJ, Nellist DJ, et al: Effects of smoking upon reproduction. *Am J Obstet Gynecol* 1966;96:267-270.
52. Peterson WF, Morese KN, Kaltreider DF: Smoking and prematurity. A preliminary report based on study of 7740 caucasians. *Obstet Gynecol* 1965;226:775-777.
53. Underwood PB, Kesler KF, O'Lane JM, et al: Parental smoking empirically related to pregnancy outcome. *Obstet Gynecol* 1967;29:1-5.

54. Yerushalmy J: Mother's cigarette smoking and survival of infant. *Am J Obstet Gynecol* 1964;88:505-509.
55. Goldstein H: Smoking in pregnancy: Some noted on the statistical controversy. *Br J Prev Soc Med* 1977;31:13-17.
56. Garn SM, Johnston M, Ridella SA, et al: The effect of maternal cigarette smoking on Apgar scores. *Am J Dis Child* 1981;135:503-506.
57. Rush D, Kass EH: Maternal smoking: A reassessment of the association with perinatal mortality. *Am J Epidemiol* 1972;96:183-196.
58. Curet LB, Vyayario A, Zachman RD, et al: Maternal smoking and respiratory distress syndrome. *Am J Obstet Gynecol* 1983;147:446-450.
59. Evans DR, Newcombe RG, Campbell H: Maternal smoking habits and congenital malformations: Population study. *Br Med J* 1979;2:171-173.
60. Ericson A, Kallen B, Westerholm P: Cigarette smoking and etiologic factors in cleft lip and palate. *Am J Obstet Gynecol* 1983;61:539-546.
61. Hemminki K, Mutanen P, Saloniemi I: Smoking and the occurrence of congenital malformations and spontaneous abortions: Multivariate analysis. *Am J Obstet Gynecol* 1983;145:61-66.
62. Naeye Rl, Peters EC: Mental development of children whose mothers smoked during pregnancy. *Obstet Gynecol* 1984;64:60-107.
63. Davie R, Butler NR, Goldstein H: *From Birth to Seven*. London, Longmans, 1972.
64. Goldstein H: Factors influencing the weight of seven year old children—results from the National Child Development Study. *Hum Biol* 1972;43:92-95.
65. Everson RB: Individuals transplacentally exposed to maternal smoking may be at increased risk in adult life. *Lancet* 1980;2:123-126.
66. Larsen CD: Pulmonary-tumor induction by transplacental exposure to urethane. *J Natl Cancer Inst* 1947;8:63-70.
67. Smith WE, Rous P: The neoplastic potentialities of mouse embryo tissues. IV. Lung adenomas in baby mice as a result of prenatal exposure to urethane. *J Exp Med* 1948;88:529-554.
68. Herbst AL, Ufelder H, Poskanzer DC: Adenocarcinoma of the vagina. Association of maternal stilbestrol therapy with tumor appearance in young women. *N Engl J Med* 1971;284:878-881.
69. Herbst AL, Scully RE, Robby SJ: Prenatal diethylstilbestrol exposure and human genital tract abnormalities. *Natl Cancer Inst Monogr* 1979;51:25-35.
70. Seeler RA, Israel JN, Royal JE, et al: Ganglioneuroblastoma and fetal hydantoin-alcohol syndromes. *Pediatrics* 1979;63:524-527.
71. Rice JM: Some overview of transplacental chemical carcinogenesis. *Teratology* 1973;8:113-126.
72. Napalkov NP: Some general considerations on the problem of transplacental carcinogenesis, in Tomatis L, Mohr U (eds): *Transplacental Carcinogenesis, IARC Sci Publ* 1973; No 4:1-13.
73. Rice JM: Perinatal period and pregnancy: Intervals of high risk for chemical carcinogens. *Environ Health Perspect* 1979;29:23-27.
74. Druckrey H, Preussmann R, Ivankovic S: N-Nitroso compounds in organotropic and transplacental carcinogenesis. *Ann NY Acad Sci* 1969;163:676-696.
75. Vesselinovitch SD: Comparative studies on perinatal carcinogenesis, in Tomatis L, Mohr U (eds): *Transplacental Carcinogenesis, IARC Sci Pub* 1973; No 4:14-22.

76. Neutel CI, Buck C: Effect of smoking during pregnancy on the risk of cancer in children. *J Natl Cancer Inst* 1971;47:59-63.
77. Gold E, Gordis L, Tonascia J, et al: Risk factors for brain tumors in children. *Am J Epidemiol* 1979;109:309-319.
78. Henderson BE, Benton B, Jing J, et al: Risk factors for cancer of the testis in young men. *Int J Cancer* 1979;23:598-602.
79. Centers for Disease Control: The fetal tobacco syndrome. *JAMA* 1985;253:2998-2999.

25 *Cigarette Smoking and Estrogen-Related Disease in Women*

John A. Baron, E. Robert Greenberg

Among the health consequences of smoking are many effects at organs lacking direct cigarette smoke contact. Although cancer in such sites can be attributed to blood-borne tobacco carcinogens, it is harder to explain other observations such as the increased risk in smokers of cardiovascular disease or adverse reproductive outcomes.

This review examines evidence that women who smoke cigarettes behave biologically as though they are estrogen-deficient.[1] Such an antiestrogenic effect of smoking could account for some of the observed health consequences which do not seem to be due to direct smoke contact. Two lines of evidence support this hypothesis. Firstly, there are epidemiologic data linking cigarette smoking to changes in the risk of estrogen-related disease, and secondly, there is experimental evidence suggesting ways in which smoking might affect production, release, and metabolism of estrogens.

EPIDEMIOLOGIC DATA

Summarized below are the epidemiologic data regarding the relationship between smoking and selected nonmalignant conditions. These include disorders related to estrogen deficiency (infertility, early natural menopause, other menstrual disorders, and osteoporosis). If smoking is associated with an antiestrogenic effect, one would expect it to increase the risk of these disorders. Also discussed is a problem that is likely to be related to estrogen excess, benign breast disease. An antiestrogenic effect of smoking might plausibly decrease the risk of this disorder.

Several of the epidemiologic reports cited below presented only scanty information on the associations with smoking. In some instances we have computed relative risks from other statistics presented in the report. In a few other instances, we have modified the summary statistics to permit comparison with those from other studies of the same topic.

Infertility

Several investigators have presented quantitative data regarding the relationship between cigarette smoking and difficulties in conceiving (Table 25-1).[2-8] Most studies, but not all, showed smokers to have a modestly decreased fertility; the positive investigations generally showed women who smoke to have a risk of infertility about 50% higher than that of comparable nonsmoking women. Three of these studies considered possible covariates in some detail, and concluded that the effect could not be attributed to other factors such as age, social class, or parity.[4,5,8] Two investigations have also demonstrated a gradient of decreasing probability of pregnancy with increasing amounts smoked,[5,8] and former smokers appear to have no impairment of fertility.[6,8] The husband's smoking history appears unrelated to fertility,[2,5] a specificity that lends support to the idea that smoking may be causally related to female infertility.

Several considerations limit the interpretation of many of the studies described above. Most did not consider separately the various types of infertility, and may have presented data for a mixture of processes. In fact, there are suggestions that smoking is primarily related to tubal infertility.[4,6,7] Similarly, studies that reported only the effects of ever-smoking may be mixing together estimates for two different exposures: current and former smoking. Most of the investigations excluded women with unplanned pregnancies, a group likely to be particularly fertile. On the other hand, several compared fertility rates only for smokers and nonsmokers who successfully became pregnant and ignored women who never conceived and whose fertility was probably most impaired. Such selection has the potential to introduce bias into the estimates of the smoking effect. Finally, information on sexual and reproductive behavior is important in assessing fertility, but only one of the studies controlled for frequency of intercourse as a potential confounding factor.[5] Thus, in view of the modest observed differences in fertility between smokers and nonsmokers, one cannot discount the possibility that bias or confounding may account for a substantial part of the effects found. Olsen et al[4] and Baird and Wilcox[5] discuss in more detail several of the artifacts that are possible.

While a negative impact of cigarette smoking on fertility is consistent with an antiestrogenic effect, other explanations have been proposed. In a comprehensive review, Mattison has discussed several possibilities, including toxic effects on ovary or sperm, and interference with implantation of the ovum.[9] The finding that tubal infertility may be the type of infertility most

Table 25-1
Cigarette Smoking and Infertility

Study	Subjects	Effect Measure	Relative Risk	Comments
Tokuhata[2]	1095 women with genital cancer; 921 with other disease	odds ratio of never having been pregnant	1.5*	no consideration of desire for pregnancy
Linn et al[3]	3214 married, non-diabetic women delivering from a planned pregnancy	probability of waiting greater than 3 months for conception	1.0	consideration only of smoking during pregnancy
Olsen el al[4]	1069 infertile women; 4305 fertile controls	odds ratio of primary infertility	1.6*	
Baird et al[5]	678 women receiving prenatal care for a planned pregnancy	fertility rate ratio	1.4*	
Daling et al[6]	159 women with tubal infertility; 159 general population women	odds ratio of tubal infertility	3.3*†	
Cramer et al[7]	283 women with tubal infertility; 3833 fertile controls	odds ratio of tubal infertility	1.6*†	
Howe el al[8]	17,032 white married women attending family planning clinics who stopped contraception	fertility rate ratio	1.3*†	effects only among heavy smokers

*Statistically significant result, $P < 0.05$.
†Derived from data presented in reference.

closely linked with smoking also suggests that nonhormonal factors might explain some of the association.

Age at Natural Menopause

The association of cigarette smoking with an early menopause is well established (Table 25-2).[10-17] In women who smoke cigarettes, natural menopause occurs between 1 and 2 years earlier than in women who do not. This has been a consistent finding in numerous studies, several of which controlled for many potentially important confounding factors.[10,14-16] The consistency of the results, and the repeated finding of a dose-response gradient, suggest

Table 25-2
Smoking and Age at Natural Menopause*

Study	Subjects	Covariates Considered	Difference in Median Age at Menopause
Jick et al[10]	2143 hospital patients	parity, marital status	1.7 yr
	1391 hospital patients	coffee/tea/alcohol consumption, hospital service, discharge patients	1.3 yr
Bailey et al[11]	733 health screening subjects	none	1.3 yr
McNamara et al[12]	1553 general population subjects	none	0.8 yr
Lindquist and Bengtsson[13]	873 general population subjects	weight	1.2 yr
Kaufman et al[14]	656 hospital patients	parity, ponderal index, age first smoked, geographic region	1.7 yr†
Adena and Gallagher[15]	10,995 health screening subjects	weight, alcohol consumption, drug taking	1.0 yr
Willett et al[16]	66,663 US nurses	height, weight, nulliparity history of hypertension or diabetes, age first smoked, time since last smoked	1.4 yr
McKinlay et al[17]	5350 general population subjects	none	1.7 yr

*Results in each study were statistically significant. Median menopausal ages for references [10,11, 13,14] were calculated by Adena and Gallagher.[16]
†Difference of mean menopausal ages.

that the association may be causal. Ex-smokers appear similar to never smokers in their age at menopause.[1]

Several mechanisms have been proposed to explain early menopause in smokers. In addition to an interference with the hypothalamic-pituitary-ovarian axis, these include a direct toxic effect on the ovary, and an alteration in the peripheral metabolism of estrogens.[1]

Other Menstrual Disorders

Several investigators have examined the relationship between smoking and menstrual problems such as dysmenorrhea, premenstrual tension, irregular menses, and secondary amenorrhea.[16-24] In every study except one,[23] cigarette smoking women reported a higher prevalence of these problems than non-smokers, though the difference was not always statistically significant. While the etiology of many of these disorders is not established, it is likely that only irregular menstruation and secondary amenorrhea might result from a relative estrogen deficiency. Four groups of investigators specifically investigated these two problems in relation to smoking.[18,19,21,22] Except for Bernhard[18] (who showed quite high risks for amenorrhea among smokers) they reported modest odds ratio elevations (between 1.1 and 1.3) for smoking women compared to never-smokers. The risk in ex-smokers was similar to that in never-smokers.

Although these findings are consistent with an association between smoking and relative estrogen deficiency, several considerations should be borne in mind. None of the four studies controlled for confounding variables in detail, and in three of them there was no control for age. Also, the similarity of these results with those for other menstrual complaints (which are probably unrelated to estrogen deficiency) suggests that some other factor associated with smoking could explain the findings.

Postmenopausal Osteoporosis

Five investigations (all case-control studies) have dealt with the effect of cigarette smoking on the risk of osteoporotic fractures in women (Table 25-3).[25-30] The four that used community controls all showed smoking to confer a substantial increase in risk.[25,26,29,30] Two of these investigations adjusted for the effects of several potential covariates such as weight. Kreiger and co-workers, however, observed only a modest increase in hip fracture risk among smoking women, and this increase was in part explained by the lean habitus of the smoking women.[27,28] This was the only study that employed hospital-

Table 25-3
Smoking and Osteoporotic Fractures

Study	Subjects	Covariates Considered	Odds Ratio
Daniell[25]	38 vertebral fracture cases 572 outpatient controls	none	4.3*
Paganini-Hill et al[26]	91 hip fracture cases; 182 retirement community controls	estrogen use, age, weight socioeconomic class, menopausal status, race, duration of residence	2.0
Kreiger et al[27,28]	98 hip fracture cases; 884 hospital controls	age, weight	1.3
Williams et al[29]	334 hip or forearm fracture cases; 567 community controls	age, habitus, estrogen use	elevated*
Aloia et al[30]	58 vertebral fracture cases; 58 healthy controls	age	3.4*

*Statistically significant result, $P < 0.05$.

ized controls. Many potential confounding variables other than weight (such as diet, alcohol use, and frequency of trauma) were not considered in any of the studies. It is possible, therefore, that some of the effect of smoking on fracture risk could be ascribed to these covariates.

Several investigators have compared bone density or mineral content in smoking and nonsmoking subjects of both sexes (Table 25-4).[25,31-39] Most of the studies of postmenopausal women have found smokers to have lower bone density than nonsmokers, but among premenopausal women there does not appear to be a difference. Lindsay[34] has presented evidence suggesting that some of the postmenopausal osteoporosis associated with smoking may be due to the lean habitus of smokers. This is supported by the epidemiologic results presented by Kreiger and co-workers,[27,28] though other investiga-

Table 25-4
Cigarette Smoking and Bone Density

Study	Subjects	Measurement Technique	Result
Daniell[25]	white, female outpatients 40-69 yrs old	cortical area	*(60-69yrs old)
Hollo et al[31]	both sexes 61-90 yrs old	single photon absorption (radius)	*
McNair et al[32]	insulin-treated diabetics both sexes, 21-70 yrs old	single photon absorption (forearm)	*
Lindquist et al[36]	general population women, 46,54,62 yrs old	dual photon absorption (lumbar spine)	†(premenopausal) §(postmenopausal)
Lindsay[34]	oophorectomized women		*(overall) §(weight-matched)
Sparrow et al[35]	healthy males, 40-80 yrs old	cortical area (hand films)	§
Rundgren and Mellstrom[36]	general population, both sexes, 70,75, 79 yrs	dual photon absorption (calcaneus)	*
Suominen et al[37]	general population men, 31-35, 51-55, 71-75 yrs old	single photon absorption (calcaneus)	*
Johnell and Nilsson[38]	general population women, 49 yrs old	single photon absorption (forearm)	†
Sowers et al[39]	general population women 55-80 yrs old	single photon absorption (radius)	†

*Statistically significant result, $P < 0.05$, with smokers' bones less dense than nonsmok[ers'].
†Smokers' bones more dense than nonsmokers'.
§Smokers' bones less dense than nonsmokers', but result not statistically significant.

tions have demonstrated an increase in the risk of fractures or osteoporosis after weight has been controlled for in analysis.[26,29,36]

Several potential mechanisms have been proposed to explain how smoking might increase the risks of osteoporotic fractures. These include various effects of chronic lung disease, as well as changes in hormones other than estrogens (eg, vitamin D, calcitonin, testosterone).[1]

Benign Breast Disease

Although the classification of benign breast disease is controversial, there is general agreement that the process is strongly related to ovarian hormones, especially estradiol and progesterone. Benign breast disease often varies in clinical severity with the menstrual cycle, and the prevalence of the problem falls off markedly after menopause.[40] Menopausal estrogens seem to exacerbate the process and several studies have documented higher levels of endogenous estrogens in cases compared to controls.[41] Benign breast disease appears to be more directly related to estrogen than does breast cancer and it is therefore a particularly interesting entity to study in attempting to link cigarette smoking with estrogen-related processes.

Berkowitz et al[42] and Pastides et al[43] and Pastides (personal communication, September 1985), both found smoking to be associated with substantially lowered risks for benign breast disease. Both groups of investigators used hospital controls and considered confounding in detail. In contrast, Nomura et al[44] did not find a consistent alteration in risk among women who smoke. Byers and his colleagues, using data from the Roswell Park Memorial Institute, have also found smoking to be unrelated to benign breast disease (personal communication, September 1985).

Berkowitz et al[42] have commented on some of the difficulties involved in case-control investigation of benign breast disease. It is likely that only a minority of women with the condition come to medical attention, and population-based controls may thus be inappropriate for comparison with a series of patients. On the other hand, any given patient control group may introduce unknown selection biases. It is possible that the divergent results in the studies cited are due to differences in case and control selection.

Summary of the Epidemiologic Data

The data summarized here are consistent with the idea that smoking women have an altered risk of estrogen-related disease. In general, cigarette smoking appears to increase the risk of estrogen-deficiency diseases (such as infertility, early menopause, and osteoporosis), and may decrease the risk of estrogen excess disease (such as endometrial cancer and benign breast disease). Ex-smokers have generally been found to be similar to never-smokers with regard to these risks, suggesting that the smoking effect is reversible after cessation of smoking. With regard to bone density and benign breast disease, premenopausal women exhibit these effects less strongly than postmenopausal women.

PHYSIOLOGICAL CONSIDERATIONS

The complexity of the female hormonal systems and the multitude of chemicals in tobacco smoke provide many opportunities for interaction. Theoretically, an antiestrogenic effect of smoking could involve any of the following:

1. Decreased production of estrogens
2. Altered metabolism of estrogens
3. Increased protein carriage of estrogens
4. Increased excretion of estrogens
5. Decreased receptor binding of estrogens
6. Non-estrogenic hormonal effects

Most of these possible mechanisms have not been investigated in detail, and only the first two will be discussed here.

Decreased Production of Estrogens

Cigarette smoke is a known ovarian toxin in rodents, and leads to ovarian atresia after chronic exposure.[9] Whether cigarette smoking is also directly toxic to the ovaries in humans is not clear, but the possibility of decreased production of estrogens in women who smoke is supported by data demonstrating decreased urinary excretion of estrogens in premenopausal smokers.[45] The epidemiologic evidence clearly indicates, however, that the effect of smoking on steroid hormones is usually reversible, while a toxic atresia of the ovaries seems unlikely to be.

A disturbance in the control of ovarian secretion is another possible way by which smoking could affect estrogen secretion. Cigarette smoking can have profound effects on the CNS including the hypothalmus, which regulates pituitary release of gonadotropins. Nicotine readily crosses the blood-brain barrier and is concentrated in the brain.[46] There are nicotine receptors throughout the nervous system; the hypothalmus is particularly well supplied with them.[47] Nicotine and cigarette smoke have been shown to enhance neurotransmission, especially in neurons using catecholamines as neurotransmitters.[48] In particular, an enhancement of dopamine turnover is thought to explain the association of nicotine or cigarette smoke exposure with low prolactin levels.[49] Dopamine also modulates LH release, and nicotine has been shown to inhibit luteinizing hormone (LH) release in rats.[49] Thus it is possible that smoking could cause a disturbance of gonadotropin release, which in turn might lead to a reversible effect on estrogen secretion and estrogenic activity.

Altered Metabolism of Estrogens

The CNS effects posited above are not relevant for postmenopausal women, since their estrogens are largely derived from adrenal sources and presumably are not under gonadotropin control. Among older women, estrogen production appears to be a generally unregulated by-product of adrenal androgen production.[50] A lack of feedback control, of course, permits greater influence by external factors. For example, steroid hormones are largely metabolized in the hepatic microsomal mixed function oxidase systems, which are induced by cigarette smoking.[51] Smokers are known to have an enhanced metabolism of certain drugs as a consequence.[52] This enzyme induction could result in an enhanced or altered metabolism of circulating estrogens which, in postmenopausal women, would not be accompanied by a compensatory change in secretion. Supporting this possibility is the observation that enzyme inducers of the type found in cigarette smoke alter the metabolism of estradiol by chick embryo hepatocytes to yield increased production of 2-hydroxyestrogens, which may have antiestrogenic properties.[53] Such an alteration in metabolism could also take place in premenopausal women, but the hypothalamic-pituitary-ovarian axis presumably could compensate for this effect in these younger age groups.

SUMMARY

A substantial body of epidemiologic evidence associates cigarette smoking with changes in the risk of estrogen-related disorders. Despite the limitations of individual studies, the results reviewed are in aggregate consistent with an antiestrogenic effect of smoking.

There is only scanty evidence regarding the metabolic processes through which smoking might affect estrogen-related disease. There are, however, a number of plausible mechanisms which provide intriguing opportunities for further laboratory studies, perhaps in conjunction with epidemiologists.

REFERENCES

1. Baron J: Smoking and estrogen-related disease. *Am J Epidemiol* 1984;119:9-22.
2. Tokuhata GK: Smoking in relation to infertility and fetal loss. *Arch Environ Health* 1968;17:353-359.
3. Linn S, Schoenbaum SC, Monson RR, et al: Delay in conception for former 'pill' users. *JAMA* 1982;247:629-632.
4. Olsen J, Rachootin P, Schiodt AV, et al: Tobacco use, alcohol consumption and infertility. *Int J Epidemiol* 1983;12:179-184.

5. Baird DD, Wilcox AJ: Cigarette smoking associated with delayed conception. *JAMA* 1985;353:2979-2983.
6. Daling JR, Weiss NS, Metch BJ, et al: Primary tubal infertility in relation to the use of an intrauterine device. *N Engl J Med* 1985;312:938-941.
7. Cramer DW, Schiff I, Schoenbaum SC, et al: Tubal infertility and the intrauterine device. *N Engl J Med* 1985;312:942-947.
8. Howe G, Westhoff C, Vessey M, et al: Effects of age, cigarette smoking and other factors on fertility: findings in a large prospective study. *Br Med J* 1985;290:1697-1700.
9. Mattison DR: The effects of smoking on fertility from gametogenesis to implantation. *Environ Res* 1982;28:410-433.
10. Jick H, Porter J, Morrison AS: Relation between smoking and age of natural menopause. *Lancet* 1977;2:1354-1355.
11. Bailey A, Robinson D, Vessey M: Smoking and age of natural menopause. *Lancet* 1977;2:722.
12. McNamara PM, Hjortland MC, Gordon T, et al: Natural history of menopause: the Framingham Study. *J Cont Ed Obstet Gynecol* 1978;20:27-35.
13. Lindlquist O, Bengtsson C: Menopausal age in relation to smoking. *Acta Med Scand* 1979;205:73-77.
14. Kaufman DW, Slone D, Rosenberg L, et al: Cigarette smoking and age at natural menopause. *Am J Public Health* 1980;70:420-422.
15. Adena MA, Gallagher HG: Cigarette smoking and the age at menopause. *Ann Hum Biol* 1982;9:121-130.
16. Willett W, Stampfer MJ, Bain C, et al: Cigarette smoking, relative weight, and menopause. *Am J Epidemiol* 1983;117:651-658.
17. McKinlay SM, Bifano NL, McKinlay JB: Smoking and age at menopause in women. *Ann Intern Med* 1985;103:350-356.
18. Bernhard VP: Sichere Schaden des Zigarettenrauchens bei der Frau. *Med Monatsschr* 1949;3:58-60.
19. Hammond EC: Smoking in relation to physical complaints. *Arch Environ Health* 1961;3:28-164.
20. Kauramiemi T: Gynecologic health screening by means of a questionnaire. *Acta Obstet Gynecol Scand* 1969;48(suppl 4):114-121.
21. Pettersson F, Fries H, Nillius SJ: Epidemiology of secondary amenorrhea. *Am J Obstet Gynecol* 1973;117:80-86.
22. Wood C: The association of psycho-social factors and gynae- cological symptoms. *Aust Fam Physician* 1978;7:471-478.
23. Andersch B, Milson I: An epidemiologic study of young women with dysmenorrhea. *Am J Obstet Gynecol* 1982;144:655-660.
24. Sloss EM, Freirichs RR: Smoking and menstrual disorders. *Int J Epidemiol* 1983;12:107-109.
25. Daniell HW: Osteoporosis of the slender smoker. *Arch Intern Med* 1976;136:298-304.
26. Paganini-Hill A, Ross RK, Gerkins VR, et al: Menopausal estrogen therapy and hip fractures. *Ann Intern Med* 1981;95:28-31.
27. Kreiger N, Kelsey JL, Holford TR, et al: An epidemiological study of hip fracture in postmenopausal women. *Am J Epidemiol* 1982;116:141-148.
28. Kreiger N, Hilditch S: Cigarette smoking and osteoporosis. *Am J Epidemiol* 1986;123:200.
29. Williams AR, Weiss NS, Ure CL: Effect of weight, smoking and estrogen use on the risk of hip and forearm fracture in postmenopausal women. *Obstet Gynecol* 1982;60:695-699.

30. Aloia JF, Cohn SH, Vaswani A, et al: Risk factors for postmenopausal osteoporosis. *Am J Med* 1985;78:95-100.
31. Hollo I, Gergely I, Boross M: Influence of heavy smoking upon the bone mineral content of the radius of the aged and effect of tobacco smoke on the sensitivity to calcitonin of rats. *Aktuel Gerontol* 1979;9:365-368.
32. McNair P, Christensen MS, Madsbad S, et al: Bone loss in patients with diabetes mellitus: effects of smoking. *Mineral Electrolyte Metab* 1980;3:94-97.
33. Lingquist O, Bengtsson C, Hansson T, et al: Bone mineral content in relation to age and menopause in middle-aged women. *Scand J Clin Lab Invest* 1981;41:215-223.
34. Lindsay R: The influence of cigarette smoking on bone mass and bone loss, in DeLuca HF, Frost HM, Jee WSS, et al (eds): *Osteoporosis: Recent Advances in Pathogenesis and Treatment.* Baltimore, University Park Press, 1981.
35. Sparrow D, Beausoleil NI, Garvey AJ, et al: The influence of cigarette smoking and age on bone loss in men. *Arch Environ Health* 1982;37:246-249.
36. Rundgren A, Mellstrom D: The effect of tobacco smoking on the bone mineral content of the ageing skeleton. *Mech Ageing Dev* 1984;28:272-277.
37. Suominen H, Heikkinen E, Vainio P, et al: Mineral density of calcaneous in men at different ages: a population study with special reference to life-style factors. *Age Ageing* 1984;13:273-281.
38. Johnell O, Nilsson BE: Life-style and bone mineral mass in perimenopausal women. *Calcif Tissue Int* 1984;35:354-356.
39. Sowers MR, Wallace RB, Lemke JH: Correlates of mid-radius bone density among postmenopausal women: a community study. *Am J Clin Nutr* 1985;41:1045-1053.
40. Cole P, Elwood JM, Kaplan SD: Incidence rates and risk factors of benign breast neoplasms. *Am J Epidemiol* 1978;108:112-120.
41. Golinger RC: Hormones and the pathophysiology of fibrocystic mastopathy. *Surg Gynecol Obstet* 1978;146:273-285.
42. Berkowitz GS, Canny PF, Livolsi VA, et al: Cigarette smoking and benign breast disease. *J Epidemiol Community* Health 1985;39:308-313.
43. Pastides H, Kelsey JF, Holford TR, et al: An Epidemiologic study of fibrocystic breast disease with reference to ductal epithelial atypia. *Am J Epidemiol* 1985;121:440-447.
44. Nomura A, Comstock GW, Tonascia JA: Epidemiologic characteristics of benign breast disease. *Am J Epidemiol* 1977;105:505-512.
45. MacMahon B, Trichopoulos D, Cole P, et al: Cigarette smoking and urinary estrogens. *N Engl J Med* 1982;307:1062-1065.
46. Sershen H, Lajtha A: Cerebral uptake of nicotine and of amino acids. *J Neurosci Res* 1979;4:65-91.
47. Morley BJ: The properties of brain nicotine receptors, in Balfour DJK (ed): *Nicotine and the Tobacco Smoking Habit.* Oxford; Pergamon Press, 1984.
48. Balfour DJK: The effects of nicotine on brain neurotransmitter systems, in Balfour DJK (ed): *Nicotine and the Tobacco Smoking Habit.* Oxford; Pergamon Press, 1984.
49. Eneroth P, Fuxe K, Gustafsson J-A: The effect of nicotine on central catecholamine neurons and gonadotropin secretion. II. Inhibitory influence of nicotine on LH, FSH, and prolactin secretion in the ovariectomized

female rat and its relation to regional changes in dopamine and noradrenaline levels and turnover. *Med Biol* 1977;55:158-166.
50. Hutton JD, Jacobs HS, James VHT: Steroid endocrinology after the menopause: a review. *J R Soc Med* 1979;72:835-841.
51. Conney AH, Pantuch EJ, Hsiao KC, et al: Regulation of drug metabolism in man by environmental chemical and diet. *Fed Proc* 1977;36:1647-1652.
52. Dawson GW, Vestal RE: Smoking and drug metabolism. *Pharmacol Ther* 1982;15:207-221.
53. Schneider J, Sassa S, Kappas A: Metabolism of estradiol in liver cell culture. *J Clin Invest* 1983;72:1420-1426.

26 *Cigarette Smoking and Endometrial Cancer*

Lynn Rosenberg, Samuel M. Lesko

Cancer of the endometrium appears to be an estrogen-related malignancy.[1] Obesity, nulliparity, older age at menopause, Stein-Leventhal syndrome, estrogen-producing tumors of the ovary, postmenopausal use of estrogen supplements, and use of sequential oral contraceptives all increase the risk; combination oral contraceptives appear to reduce it. These associations are explicable, at least in part, by exposure of the endometrium to unopposed estrogen of either endogenous or exogenous origin.

MacMahon et al[2] found that urinary levels of the three major endogenous estrogens were lower for smokers than for nonsmokers during the luteal phase of the menstrual cycle. If the reduced levels in smokers also reflect a reduction in stimulation of the endometrium by estrogen, then it may be that the incidence of endometrial cancer is reduced in smokers.

The results of previous studies[3-9] on the relation of endometrial cancer risk to cigarette smoking have been inconclusive (Table 26-1). In the case-control studies of Williams and Horm,[3] Weiss et al,[4] Kelsey et al,[5] and Tyler et al,[6] the risk of endometrial cancer appeared lower in smokers than in nonsmokers, but only in the study of Weiss et al was the reduction statistically significant. The data of two of the studies suggested that an effect of smoking may be confined to older or postmenopausal women. In particular, Tyler et al studied women aged 20 to 54 years: the relative risk estimate was 1.1 in premeno-pausal women versus 0.8 in postmenopausal women, and it was 1.1 among women who were less than 50 years old versus 0.7 among women aged 50-54 years.[6] In the study of Weiss et al in which

Table 26-1
Cigarette Smoking and Endometrial Cancer

Study	Subjects	Confounding Factors Considered	Contrast	Event	Relative Risks
Case-control					
Williams and Horm[3]	358 cases, 3189 controls with other cancers	Age, race	<20 pack-years 20-40 pack-years ≥40 pack-years *v* never-smoker	Incidence	0.9 0.8 0.7
Weiss et al[4]	322 cases, 289 community controls	Age, parity, weight, hypertension, estrogen use	Ever- *v* never-smoker	Incidence	0.4*
Kelsey et al[5]	167 cases, 903 hospital controls	Age, parity, weight, menopausal status, education, OC/estrogen use, and others	Ever-regular *v* never-smoker	Incidence	0.8†
Tyler et al[6]	437 cases, 3200 community controls	Age, weight, OC use, alcohol use, menopausal status, estrogen use	Ever *v* never, Current *v* never-smoker	Incidence	0.9 0.8
Follow-up					
Cederlof et al[7]	27,732 women 80 cases, 33 deaths	age	Current *v* never-smoker	Incidence, death	0.7† 1.9†
Garfinkel[8]	375,381 women 224 deaths	age	Regular smoker *v* entire cohort	Death	1.0

*$P < 0.05$.
†As derived by Baron.[9]

there was a statistically significant effect of smoking, the women studied were at least 50 years old.[4] There have been two follow-up studies with data on the incidence of endometrial cancer according to smoking status,[7-8] but since neither contained information on the prevalence of hysterectomy, the results are difficult to interpret.

In the present report the results of a case-control study of endometrial cancer and cigarette smoking recently completed by the Drug Epidemiology Unit (DEU) are discussed.[10]

METHODS

The DEU data were obtained in a case-control study conducted from 1976 to 1983 in medical centers located chiefly on the eastern seaboard of the United States.[10] Information was collected by interview of women with endometrial cancer (cases) and women with other selected malignancies (controls). Women admitted for endometrial cancer diagnosed no more than 6 months previously, who were 30 to 69 years of age, who had no history of a previous or concurrent malignancy, and who had not had a bilateral oophorectomy constituted the case series (510 women). The controls (727 women) had been admitted for colorectal cancer (291), malignant melanoma (279), or lymphorecticular malignancies or cancer of the thyroid or adrenal glands (157), none of which had been diagnosed more than 6 months previously. Like the cases, the controls were 30 to 69 years of age, had no history of a previous or concurrent malignancy, had an intact uterus, and had not had a bilateral oophorectomy.

RESULTS

Table 26-2 gives the smoking habits of the cases and controls. For current smokers (women who had smoked in the previous year) relative to women who had never smoked, the estimated relative risk (RR) of endometrial cancer was 0.7 (95% confidence interval [CI] = 0.5-1.0) after allowance for age, body mass index (weight/height^2), and conjugated estrogen use.[11,12] For current smokers of one to 14 cigarettes per day and 15 to 24 cigarettes per day, the estimates were compatible with 1.0, while for smokers of 25 or more cigarettes daily, the relative risk estimate was significantly below unity: RR = 0.5 (CI = 0.3-0.8). For former smokers (women who had last smoked at least 1 year previously), the overall relative risk estimate was 0.9 (CI = 0.6-1.2). In addition, the estimates for categories of the number of cigarettes per day last smoked among ex-smokers were all close to unity (not shown). There were insufficient data to permit informative analysis of the relation of the risk of endometrial cancer to the duration of the interval since cessation of smoking.

To allow for all identified potential confounding factors, multiple logistic regression analyses were carried out.[13] Allowance was made for the follow-

Table 26-2
Cigarette Use Among 510 Cases of Endometrial Cancer and 727 Controls

Smoking Status	Cases		Controls		Relative Risk Estimate* (95% Confidence Interval)	
Never smoked	282	(55)†	335	(47)	1.0§	
Former smoker	113	(22)	161	(23)	0.9	(0.6-1.2)
Current smoker (cigarettes/d)						
1-14	36	(7)	51	(7)	0.8	(0.5-1.3)
15-24	49	(10)	85	(11)	1.0	(0.6-1.5)
≥25	28	(5)	74	(9)	0.5	(0.3-0.8)

Data from Drug Epidemiology Unit Study[10]; two cases and 21 controls with unknown smoking status are not included.
*Mantel-Haenszel estimate calculated from data stratified by age, body mass index, and duration of conjugated estrogen use.
†Numbers in parentheses are percentages standardized to the age distribution of the cases.
§Reference category.

ing factors: age, race, religion, years of education, body mass index, history of drug-treated diabetes mellitus, history of drug-treated hypertension, age at first pregnancy, parity, menopausal status, age at menopause, history of removal of one ovary, history of cholecystectomy, conjugated estrogen use, oral contraceptive use, alcohol use, number of previous hospital admissions, geographic area, and year of interview. Estimates so obtained were not materially different from those already presented.

In Table 26-3, data on women who had never smoked or who were current smokers of 25 or more cigarettes daily are divided according to menopausal status. The relative risk estimate for smokers of 25 or more cigarettes daily was significantly below 1.0 in postmenopausal women (RR = 0.5, CI – 0.2-0.9) and close to unity in premenopausal women (RR = 0.9, CI = 0.4-2.2), but the two estimates did not differ significantly from each other. The data for postmenopausal women were further divided according to the age at reaching menopause (not shown): within each category, the relative risk estimate for smokers of 25 or more cigarettes daily was below 1.0, but confidence intervals were wide.

Obese women, nulliparous women, and those who use conjugated estrogens are at increased risk of endometrial cancer.[1] Data on smoking according to categories of these factors are given in Table 26-4. The relative risk estimates for current smokers of 25 or more cigarettes daily were below unity in all categories of body mass index, among nulliparous as well as among parous women, and among estrogen users as well as among women who did

Table 26-3
Cigarette Use Among 510 Cases of Endometrial Cancer and 727 Controls by Menopausal Status

Status	Cigarette Use	Cases	Controls	Relative Risk Estimate (95% Confidence Interval)
Premenopausal	Never smoked	42	152	1.0†
	≥25 cigarettes/d	8	38	0.9 (0.4-2.2)
Postmenopausal	Never smoked	233	179	1.0†
	≥25 cigarettes/d	20	34	0.5 (0.2-0.9)

Data from the Drug Epidemiology Unit study[10]; limited to current smokers of a least 25 cigarettes per day or women who had never smoked.
*Mantel-Haenszel estimate calculated from data stratified by age, body mass index and duration of conjugated estrogen use.
†Reference category.

not use estrogens. Most of the estimates, however, were not statistically significant.

DISCUSSION

The results presented here, taken with previous evidence, suggest that the incidence of endometrial cancer is lower in women who smoke than in those who have never smoked. There are still insufficient data to establish the details of the relation between endometrial cancer and smoking. For example, it has not been established whether the risk is related to the amount smoked. Among ex-smokers, it is not known whether the risk returns to baseline with progressively longer intervals after cessation of smoking.

The relation between endometrial cancer and smoking may be stronger in postmenopausal women than in premenopausal women, or even present only in postmenopausal women. One possible explanation is that an antiestrogenic effect of smoking in premenopausal women might be small relative to the protective effect of endogenous progesterone, whereas in postmenopausal women, an effect might be more apparent because of the relative paucity of progesterone.

The present data also suggest that a reduction in the risk of endometrial cancer occurs among smokers who are otherwise at increased risk because of taking estrogen supplements; this was also the case in the study of Weiss et al.[4] In addition, the DEU results suggest that the effect is independent of body mass index or parity. The data on these subgroups are scanty, however, and larger studies are needed to assess whether a relation between endometrial cancer and smoking is modified by these and other factors.

Finally, if smoking does indeed reduce the risk of endometrial cancer, this does not have any direct public health importance, since the magnitude of

Table 26-4
Cigarette Use Among 510 Cases of Endometrial Cancer and 727 Controls by Body Mass Index, Parity, and Conjugated Estrogen Use

Factor	Cigarette Use	Cases	Controls	Relative Risk Estimates (95% Confidence Interval)
Body mass index*				
≥30	Never smoked	91	52	1.0†
	≥25 cigarettes/d	5	10	0.4 (0.2-1.0)
24-29	Never smoked	96	98	1.0†
	≥25 cigarettes/d	10	22	0.7 (0.3-1.6)
<24	Never smoked	85	177	1.0†
	≥25 cigarettes/d	13	39	0.5 (0.2-1.2)
Parity				
0	Never smoked	59	69	1.0†
	≥25 cigarettes/d	7	13	0.7 (0.3-2.1)
1-3	Never smoked	162	198	1.0†
	≥25 cigarettes/d	17	48	0.7 (0.2-0.9)
≥4	Never smoked	49	61	1.0†
	≥25 cigarettes/d	2	10	0.4 (0.1-2.9)
Conjugated Estrogen Use				
≥1 yr	Never smoked	78	16	1.0†
	≥25 cigarettes/d	10	4	0.8 (0.2-3.5)
Never used	Never smoked	197	315	1.0†
	≥25 cigarettes/d	17	68	0.5 (0.3-0.8)

Data from Drug Epidemiology Unit Study[10]; limited to current smokers of at least 25 cigarettes per day and women who had never smoked.
*Weight (kg)/height^2 (cm); Mantel-Haenszel relative risk estimates calculated from data stratified by age and duration of conjugated estrogen use.
†Reference categories. Mantel-Haenszel relative risk estimate calculated from data stratified by age, body mass index, and duration of conjugated estrogen use.

the adverse effects of smoking on health far outweighs any potential benefits. Elucidation of how smoking reduces the risk, however, could well shed light on how endometrial cancer is caused.

Acknowledgments

This work was supported by contracts 223-76-3016, 223-80-3001, 226-82-0007 from the Food and Drug Administration, contracts NO1-CP-71029 and NO1-CB-74099 from the National Cancer Institute, contract NO1-HD-02810 from the National Institute of Child Health and Human Development, and by a grant-in-aid from Hoffmann-La Roche Inc, Nutley, NJ. The Drug Epidemiology Unit also receives support from Ciba-Geigy Corp, Summit, NJ; Hoechst AG, Frankfurt, West Germany; McNeil Pharmaceutical, Springhouse, Pa; Merrell Dow Pharmaceuticals, Inc, Cincinnati; General Foods Corp, White Plains, NY; Ortho Pharmaceutical Corp, Raritan, NJ; the National Coffee Association of USA, Inc; and the Alcoholic Beverage Medical Research Foundation, Baltimore.

REFERENCES

1. Kelsey JL, Hildreth NG: *Breast and Gynecologic Cancer Epidemiology.* Boca Raton, CRC Press, 1983.
2. MacMahon B, Trichopoulos D, Cole P, et al: Cigarette smoking and urinary estrogens. *N Engl J Med* 1982;307:1062-1065.
3. Williams RR, Horm JW: Association of cancer sites with tobacco and alcohol consumption and socioeconomic status of patients: interview study from the Third National Cancer Survey. *J Natl Cancer Inst* 1977;58:525-547.
4. Weiss NS, Farewell VT, Szekely DR, et al: Oestrogens and endometrial cancer: effect of other risk factors on the association. *Maturitas* 1980;2:185-190.
5. Kelsey JL, LiVolsi, Holford TR, et al: A case-control study of cancer of the endometrium. *Am J Epidemiol* 1982;116:333-342.
6. Tyler CW, Webster LA, Ory HW, et al: Endometrial cancer: How does cigarette smoking influence the risk of women under 55 years having this tumor? *Am J Obstet Gynecol* 1985;151:899-905.
7. Cederlof R, Friberg L, Hrubec Z, et al: *The Relationship of Smoking and Some Social Covariables to Mortality and Cancer Morbidity.* Stockholm, Dept of Environmental Hygiene, Karolinska Institute, 1975.
8. Garfinkel L: Cancer mortality in non-smokers: prospective study of the American Cancer Society. *J Natl Cancer Inst* 1980;65:1169-1173.
9. Baron JA: Smoking and estrogen-related disease. *Am J Epidemiol* 1984;19:9-22.
10. Lesko SM, Rosenberg L, Kaufman DW, et al: Cigarette smoking and endometrial cancer. *N Engl J Med* 1985;313:593-596.
11. Mantel H, Haenzel W: Statistical aspects of the analysis of data from retrospective studies. *J Natl Cancer Inst* 1959;22:719-748.
12. Miettinen OS: Estimability and estimation in case referent studies. *Am J Epidemiol* 1976;103:226-235.
13. Armitage P: *Statistical Methods in Medical Research.* New York, John Wiley & Sons, 1971.

27 *Cigarette Smoking and Breast Cancer*

Nancy E. Stroup, Peter M. Layde, Linda A. Webster, Phyllis A. Wingo, George L. Rubin, Howard W. Ory, and The Cancer and Steroid Hormone Study Group

About a third of American women smoke cigarettes.[1] Since women lagged behind men by 25 to 30 years in the onset of widespread cigarette use, the impact of smoking-related diseases on the health of women is just now becoming apparent. The increase in smoking among women since World War II has been followed by a dramatic increase in mortality from lung cancer (Figure 27-1).[2] Between 1960 and 1982, mortality rates from breast cancer were nearly stable, while mortality rates from lung cancer increased more than fourfold. Lung cancer has recently overtaken breast cancer to become the leading cause of cancer mortality among American women.

Data do not suggest that breast cancer mortality is strongly related to smoking habits (Figure 27-1), but smoking could have a modest effect on breast cancer risk. In fact, it has recently been proposed that smoking might

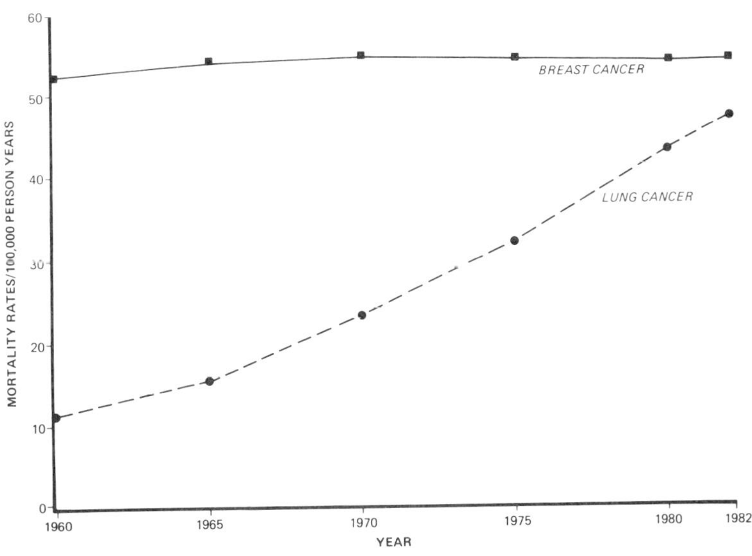

Figure 27-1 Breast and lung cancer mortality rates among women aged 35-84 years in the United States (adjusted to the age distribution of the total population in 1942[2]).

decrease the risk of breast cancer. In a 1982 study, MacMahon et al found that premenopausal women who smoked cigarettes had lower urinary estrogen levels than those who did not smoke.[3] They suggested that a decrease in estrogen levels due to smoking might lead to a decreased risk of breast cancer. Vessey et al[4] found some support for this hypothesis in 1983. In their hospital-based case-control study, they found that breast cancer risk was 23% lower in women who smoked one to 14 cigarettes per day than in women who never smoked. Prompted by this finding, Baron[5] reviewed previous studies of the effects of smoking on a variety of diseases thought to be affected by estrogen levels. For conditions such as age at menopause, osteoporosis, and uterine cancer, the review suggested that smoking could have an antiestrogenic effect, but the findings were inconsistent with regard to the risk of breast cancer among smokers. Baron identified studies in which there was a positive association, a negative association, and no association between breast cancer risk and smoking. The range in the reported effects was modest, however, with most risk-ratio estimates in the range of 0.8-1.2. In an analysis of a hospital-based case-control study reported in 1984, Rosenberg et al[6] found that, compared with "never-smokers", the relative risk of breast cancer was 1.1 in current smokers and 1.0 in those who smoked 15 or more cigarettes per day. In summary, findings from epidemiologic studies of the relationship between breast cancer risk and smoking have been inconsistent. The results suggest, however, that if smoking influences the risk of breast cancer, the effect is quite modest.

We examined the association between smoking and breast cancer, using data from a large population-based case-control study. This study, known as the Cancer and Steroid Hormone Study, is coordinated by the Division of Reproductive Health at the Centers for Disease Control, with support from the National Institute for Child Health and Development and the National Cancer Institute. This study is well suited for examining the relationship between smoking and breast cancer for two reasons. First, the estimate of smoking prevalence among the controls was obtained from a sample of the general population, rather than from a hospital-based control group. Since smoking causes or aggravates many conditions that lead to hospitalization, prevalence estimates derived from a hospital-based group could be artificially high, leading to a biased estimate of the relative risk. Second, previous studies have suggested that if smoking does alter the risk of breast cancer, the risk is quite small. Since over 9000 breast cancer cases and controls are included in the Cancer and Steroid Hormone Study, these risk ratios can be estimated with greater precision than in previous studies.

The methods used in this study have been reported elsewhere.[7] In brief, breast cancer cases and controls were ascertained over a 2-year period from eight areas in the United States where population-based information on cancer incidence is collected. Women who lived in these areas were included as cases if they had histologically confirmed primary breast cancer and if they were between 20 and 54 years of age at the time of diagnosis. Control women were selected by random telephone dialing in these eight areas. Control women were frequency matched to the 5-year age distribution of the cases and were excluded if they had a previous history of breast cancer. Information on reproduction patterns, use of contraceptives, and personal characteristics was obtained with a standardized questionnaire administered to the participants in their homes. Since the primary focus of the study was to examine the relationship between breast cancer and oral contraceptive use, women over 54 years of age at the time of diagnosis were not included in this study, because they had little opportunity to use oral contraceptives during their reproductive years.

Smoking status was ascertained initially by asking women if they had smoked 100 or more cigarettes in their lifetimes. Those who said "yes" were asked when they began smoking, the average number of cigarettes smoked per day, whether they smoked continuously or intermittently, and when they had last smoked. Women were considered current smokers if they had been smoking less than 1 year before diagnosis or interview. Included in this analysis were 4720 women with breast cancer and 4682 control women. Only 13 of the available women were excluded because their smoking histories were inadequate.

Odds ratios were calculated as estimates of relative risk (RR) by using both the Mantel-Haenszel method and unconditional logistic regression, and 95% confidence intervals (CIs) were calculated for both types of estimates. To assess the effects of potentially confounding variables on the estimate of risk, we included the following risk factors for breast cancer in logistic regression analyses: age at diagnosis or interview, age at first full-term pregnancy, parity, adiposity (as measured by Quetelet's index), family history of breast cancer, history of benign breast disease, menopausal status, oral contraceptive use, and postmenopausal estrogen use. Analyses were also done to assess whether any of these risk factors modified the association between smoking and breast cancer.

The crude relative risks and relative risks were adjusted for the effects of potentially confounding variables (Table 27-1). A very slight increase in breast cancer risk was found for both current and former smokers, compared with women who never smoked. The crude relative risk for breast cancer is 1.1 among current smokers, and the adjusted relative risk is 1.2. For former smokers, the crude relative risk is 1.2, and the adjusted relative risk is 1.1. Since the crude and adjusted risk ratios are nearly the same, the risk estimates are not influenced by the potentially confounding factors included in the logistic model. The adjusted relative risks (Table 27-2) indicate that for both current and former smokers there is no strong association between breast cancer and the age at which women first smoked, the average number of cigarettes smoked per day, the total number of years they smoked, or the number of years since they first smoked (latency). The risk estimates (Table 27-2) range

Table 27-1
Risk Ratios for Breast Cancer Among Current and Ex-Smokers

Smoking Status	Cases (n=4720)	Controls (n=4682)	RR_c	RR_a	95% CI of RR_a
Never	43%	46%	1.0	1.0	Referent
Current	39%	38%	1.1	1.2	1.0-1.3
Ex-smokers*	18%	16%	1.2	1.1	1.0-1.3

RR_c = Crude risk ratio; RR_a = risk ratio adjusted for the effects of potentially confounding variables (age at diagnosis or interview, age at first full-term pregnancy, parity, adiposity [Quetelet's index], family history of breast cancer, history of benign breast disease, menopausal status, oral contraceptive use, and postmenopausal estrogen use); CI = 95% confidence interval.
*Stopped smoking >1 year before diagnosis or interview.

from 1.0 to 1.3, and no consistent relationship was found between breast cancer risk and any smoking characteristic. Since dose-response effects were not found, it seems unlikely that smoking actually increases breast cancer risk. The slight elevations in risk could be an artifact due to differential reporting of smoking histories by cases and controls, or they could reflect the residual

Table 27-2
Adjusted Risk Ratios for Breast Cancer by Smoking Characteristics (Referent = Never-Smokers)

Smoking Characteristics	Current Smokers		Ex-Smokers	
	RR_a	95% CI	RR_a	95% CI
Age first smoked (yr)				
<15	1.1	0.9-1.4	1.2	0.8-1.7
15-19	1.1	1.0-1.3	1.1	0.9-1.3
≥20	1.2	1.0-1.4	1.3	0.9-1.4
Average no. of cigarettes smoked per day				
<15	1.1	1.0-1.3	1.1	0.9-1.3
15-24	1.2	1.0-1.3	1.1	0.9-1.3
≥25	1.2	1.0-1.4	1.3	1.0-1.7
Total no. of years smoked				
<15	1.1	0.9-1.3	1.1	0.9-1.3
15-29	1.2	1.0-1.3	1.2	1.0-1.5
≥30	1.1	1.0-1.3	1.0	0.7-1.7
No. of years since first smoked				
<15	1.1	0.9-1.4	1.1	0.8-1.5
15-29	1.2	1.0-1.3	1.1	1.0-1.3
≥30	1.1	1.0-1.3	1.1	0.9-1.3

For abbreviations, see footnote to Table 27-1.
*Stopped smoking >1 year before diagnosis or interview.

Table 27-3
Adjusted Risk Ratios for Breast Cancer Among Current and Never-Smokers by Postmenopausal Estrogen Use

	Smoking Status			
Postmenopausal Estrogen Use	Never RR_a	95% CI	Current RR_a	95% CI
Never	1.0	Referent	1.2	1.1-1.3
Ever	1.1	0.8-1.5	0.8	0.5-1.1*

For abbreviations, see footnote to Table 27-1.
**P*-value for current smoker: postmenopausal estrogen interaction is .02.

effects of other, unmeasured factors, such as nutritional status, that could increase breast cancer risk.

We also assessed whether the association between breast cancer and smoking was modified by known risk factors for breast cancer. This analysis was restricted to current and never-smokers. Our analysis suggested that the effect of smoking was modified slightly by one variable, postmenopausal estrogen use. Women who were current smokers and who took postmenopausal estrogens had an adjusted relative risk for breast cancer of 0.8 (Table 27-3); those who were current smokers but did not take postmenopausal estrogens had a relative risk of 1.2. This modest association should be interpreted with caution, since many comparisons were made in this analysis. Furthermore, this finding is puzzling in that the overall association between postmenopausal estrogen use and breast cancer risk was not significantly elevated in this study. Only 1.7% of the women with breast cancer in this study both smoked and took postmenopausal estrogens, so the overall public health impact of the decreased risk, if it is a real effect, is quite small. It would be useful if the relationship between smoking, estrogen use, and breast cancer could be addressed by using data from other epidemiologic studies, particularly those that include women over 54 years of age.

In summary, we found that, for women 20 to 54 years of age, risk of breast cancer was slightly elevated among both current and former smokers. Since a dose-response effect was not found between breast cancer risk and various characteristics of smokers, we concluded that the slightly increased risk could well be an artifact due to biases inherent in observational studies. We also found some evidence of a decreased breast cancer risk among women who both smoked and took postmenopausal estrogens. If this association is real, then it is consistent with the hypothesis that smoking has a modest antiestrogenic effect.

Studies of the effect of cigarette smoke on estrogen levels may provide some insight into the etiology of breast cancer and other hormonally mediated conditions. Our most important goal, however, is to convince women of all ages that they should not smoke. The health hazards of smoking are substantial for women and their offspring, and any benefit that might be related to an antiestrogenic effect of cigarette smoke is inconsequential compared with these hazards.

Acknowledgments

Supported by interagency agreement 3-Y01-HD-8-1037 between the Centers for Disease Control and the National Institute of Child Health and Human Development, with additional support from the National Cancer Institute.

REFERENCES

1. Remington PO, Forman MR, Gentry EM, et al: Current smoking trends in the U.S.: the 1981-1983 Behavioral Risk Factor Survey. *JAMA* 1985;253: 2975-2978.
2. Mortality trends of lung and breast cancer in women. *Stat Bull Metrop Insur Co* 1985;66:4-9.
3. MacMahon B, Trichopoulos D, Cole P, et al: Cigarette smoking and urinary estrogens. *N Engl J Med* 1982;307:1062-1065.
4. Vessey M, Baron J, Doll R, et al: Oral contraceptives and breast cancer: final report of an epidemiologic study. *Br J Cancer* 1983;47:455-462.
5. Baron JA: Smoking and estrogen-related disease. *Am J Epidemiol* 1984;119:9-22.
6. Rosenberg L, Schwingi PJ, Kaufman D, et al: Breast cancer and cigarette smoking. *N Engl J Med* 1984;310:92-94.
7. Centers for Disease Control Cancer and Steroid Hormone Study: Long-term oral contraceptive use and the risk of breast cancer. *JAMA* 1983;249:1591-1595.

28 *Smoking and Epithelial Ovarian Cancer*

Adele L. Franks

Ovarian cancer is the fifth leading cause of cancer death among women. Because of difficulty in detecting and in treating this cancer, it has a very poor prognosis. Although the causes of ovarian cancer are not understood, several mechanisms have been proposed, each of which may be affected by cigarette smoking.

Two hypotheses of epithelial ovarian carcinogenesis arose from the consistent findings that parity and oral contraceptive use are each associated with a reduced risk of ovarian cancer. One hypothesis to explain this finding is that repeated ovulation, by continually disrupting the ovarian epithelium, leads to malignant transformation, and that interrupting ovulation by pregnancy or oral contraceptive use stops this process in some way. The second hypothesis is that gonadotropin stimulation of the ovary may play a causative role in carcinogenesis and that pregnancy and oral contraceptives may be protective because both decrease circulating gonadotropins. The third hypothesis is that carcinogens in the local environment of the ovary contribute to the development of this cancer.

Each of these proposed mechanisms can be influenced by cigarette smoking. It is well established that smokers have earlier menopause,[1-3] and there is some evidence of decreased fertility.[4,5] Therefore it is possible that smokers have fewer lifetime ovulations than nonsmokers. If ovulation is the primary mechanism of ovarian carcinogenesis one might therefore expect that cigarette smokers would be at a decreased risk of ovarian cancer compared to nonsmokers. However, by the gonadotropin stimulation theory the opposite might be expected. As Baron[6] clearly illustrates, smoking is associated with diminished estrogen status. The pituitary gland may reflexively release more gonadotropins in response to decreased circulating estrogens in smokers, leading to an increased risk of ovarian cancer. Lastly, if carcinogens which are known to be present in the circulatory systems, urine, and cervical mucus of smokers are also present in the local vicinity of the ovary, one might expect that smokers would be at increased risk of ovarian cancer compared with nonsmokers. Therefore, from the prevailing hypotheses of ovarian carcinogenesis it is reasonable to expect that smoking might affect a woman's risk of developing ovarian cancer, and also that analysis of this issue might help elucidate the mechanisms of ovarian carcinogenesis.

Some previous studies of ovarian cancer have incidentally reported on the risks associated with smoking, but none have systematically studied this question in detail. In 1966 Hammond[7] compared death rates of smokers and nonsmokers for a variety of diseases. For ovarian cancer, the mortality ratio of smokers compared to nonsmokers was 0.99 while for heavier smokers it was 1.15. A follow-up study of over 6000 female British physicians, reported by Doll et al[8] in 1980, found a significant elevation in ovarian cancer death rates for smokers versus nonsmokers, but no direct relationship of death rate with amount smoked.

Of the case-control studies that provide any information on the association of smoking with ovarian cancer, none report a statistically significant association. Byers et al[9] included smoking in a hospital-based study of dietary and nondietary risk factors, and found an age-adjusted relative risk estimate of 0.9 for ever-smokers compared with never smokers. Cramer et al[10] reported a population-based study of dietary risk factors which found a relative risk estimate of 1.8 for smokers versus nonsmokers which was not statistically significant. They also found no significant trend of risk in relation to lifetime dose (in pack-years) of cigarette smoking. Mori et al[11] reported no significant difference in the use of tobacco between their cases and controls although no numbers were given. Similarly a hospital-based study by Tzonou et al[12] found relative risks of 1.1 for light smokers and 0.8 for heavier smokers.

Thus, from the literature on the subject to date, there is no evidence of a significant effect of smoking on ovarian cancer. However, none of these studies examined the issue in depth and none controlled for factors that could camouflage an association. For example, age is associated with an increased risk of developing epithelial ovarian cancer, while parity and oral contraceptive use are associated with a decreased risk. Unless statistical adjustment is made for these factors, findings could be distorted. None of the previous studies have controlled for all three of these important potential confounding factors. Therefore the possibility of a masking of an association remains a concern.

To systemically evaluate the effect of cigarette smoking on epithelial ovarian cancer, data from the Cancer and Steroid Hormone Study is being analyzed. This is a population-based case-control study of ovarian, breast, and endometrial cancers. We are comparing women with epithelial ovarian cancer to controls with regard to ever having smoked cigarettes, recency of smoking, cumulative lifetime dose of cigarette smoking (in pack-years), time since beginning to smoke, and age at which smoking started.[13] Preliminary analysis of approximately 400 cases and 4000 controls shows no effect of any of these smoking variables on the risk of developing epithelial ovarian cancer. Even when simultaneously adjusting for age, parity, prior oral contraceptive use, and other potential confounders by logistic regression techniques, no effects of smoking are detectable (Table 28-1, preliminary data).

Thus, despite theoretical predictions, there appears to be no indication that smoking appreciably influences the development of epithelial ovarian cancer. Of course, this should not be reassuring to smokers who suffer sub-

Table 28-1
Risk of Epithelial Ovarian Cancer by Pack-years of Cigarette Smoking (preliminary results)

Pack-years	Cases	Controls	Relative Risk*	95% Confidence Interval
Never smoked	201	1718	1.0	Referent
Ever smoked				
<5	47	497	0.8	(0.6-1.1)
5-9	28	264	0.9	(0.6-1.4)
10-19	54	489	1.0	(0.7-1.4)
20-29	47	353	1.3	(0.9-1.8)
30-39	37	276	1.1	(0.8-1.7)
≥40	30	243	1.2	(0.8-1.8)

*Adjusted for age, parity, oral contraceptive use.

stantially increased morbidity and mortality from other diseases attributable to cigarette smoking. But it does appear that even in a smoke-free society we may still be confronted with the challenge to better understand and eventually prevent ovarian cancer.

REFERENCES

1. Jick H, Porter J, Morrison AS: Relation between smoking and age of natural menopause. *Lancet* 1977;1:1354-1155.
2. Kaufman DW, Slone D, Rosenberg L, et al: Cigarette smoking and age at natural menopause. *Am J Public Health* 1980;70:420-422.
3. Willett W, Stampfer MJ, Bain C, et al: Cigarette smoking, relative weight, and menopause. *Am J Epidemiol* 1983;117:651-658.
4. Baird DD, Wilcox AJ: Cigarette smoking associated with delayed conception. *JAMA* 1985;253:2979-2983.
5. Olsen J, Rachootin P, Schiodt AV, et al: Tobacco use, alcohol consumption and infertility. *Int J Epidemiol* 1982;12:179-184.
6. Baron JA: Smoking and estrogen-related disease. *Am J Epidemiol* 1984;119:9-22.
7. Hammond EC: Smoking in relation to death rates of one million men and women. *Natl Cancer Inst Monogr* 1966;19:127-204.
8. Doll R, Gray R, Hafner B, et al: Mortality in relation to smoking: 22 years' observations on female British doctors. *Br Med J* 1980;280(6219):967-971.
9. Byers T, Marshall J, Graham S, et al: A case-control study of dietary and nondietary factors in ovarian cancer. *J Natl Cancer* Inst 1983;71:681-686.
10. Cramer DW, Welch WR, Hutchinson GB, et al: Dietary animal fat in relation to ovarian cancer risk. *Obstet Gynecol* 1984;63:833-838.
11. Mori M, Kiyosawa H, Miyake H: Case-control study of ovarian cancer in Japan. *Cancer* 1984;53:2746-2752.
12. Tzonou A, Day NE, Trichopoulos D, et al: The epidemiology of ovarian cancer in Greece: a case-control study. *Eur J Cancer Clin Oncol* 1984;20:1045-1052.
13. The Centers for Disease Control Cancer and Steroid Hormone Study: Long-term oral contraceptive use and the risk of breast cancer: *JAMA* 1983;249:1591-1595

29 *Smoking and Cervical Cancer*

Shanna Swan

Since 1966, when Naguib et al[1] demonstrated that current smokers had an increased risk of carcinoma in situ, the question of a possible etiologic role for cigarette smoking in cervical intraepithelial neoplasia has been frequently studied and debated. In this paper the available literature on this subject will be reviewed and summarized in an attempt to assess the likelihood that this association is a causal one. Studies will be evaluated as to the appropriateness of control selection, the adequacy of sample size, and the control of principal confounders, including sexual behavior and oral contraceptive (OC) use. Recent laboratory data, which have suggested some possible mechanisms of action, will also be summarized.

HISTORICAL REVIEW

Between 1966 and 1977, a number of studies were published containing data that could be analyzed to examine the relationship between smoking and cervical neoplasia (Table 29-1).[2-7] These data were not collected to address the smoking-cervical cancer hypothesis, however, and the important confounders for this association were not considered. None of these studies controlled for sexual behavior and few for OC use. Nevertheless, all relative risk estimates for smoking were reported to be above 1.0, and several studies demonstrated a modest dose-response relationship.[3,4,6]

In 1977, Winkelstein[8] hypothesized a causal relationship between smoking and squamous cervical cancer, prompted by the ecological correlation between age-adjusted incidence rates for cervical cancer and lung cancer in the Third National Cancer Survey and by the observation that the association between smoking and lung cancer is found predominantly in squamous cell tumors. He noted that this hypothesis was consistent with published data from a number of sources.[1,2,4,7]

In the next few years, three studies provided additional information on this issue.[9-11] Like the earlier studies, these had not been designed to address the smoking and cervical cancer hypothesis. However, two studies[9,10] provided evidence of a dose-response relationship for each of three levels of severity of cervical neoplasia. Wright et al[9] noted that smoking was found to be a major risk factor, after the data were adjusted for contraception and sexual behavior, as measured by age at first coitus and number of sexual partners. Nevertheless, the authors concluded that this relationship "probably implies that the smoking habit reflects some important aspects of sexual behavior relevant to the production of disease that we have been unable to measure."

Table 29-1
Studies Not Designed to Test Smoking-Cervical Cancer Hypothesis

Author (Year)	Case Definition	Smoking Comparison	Relative Risk Estimate
Naguib et al (1966)[1]	Preinvasive	Current *v* never	2.1
Thomas (1973)[2]	In situ	"Regular" *v* never	1.7
Kessler et al (1974)[3]	Invasive	Current *v* never (Moslems)	2.6
		21+ *v* never	5.0
		Current *v* never (non-Moslems)	1.2
		21+ *v* never	1.2
Cederlof et al (1975)[4]	"Registered"	1-15 *v* never	2.9
		15+ *v* never	3.4
Hirayama (1975)[5]	Deaths	Daily *v* "nonsmoker"	1.7
Williams and Horm (1977)[7]	Invasive	1-20 pack-years *v* never	1.2
		20-40 pack years *v* never	1.6
		>40 pack years *v* never	1.8
Peritz et al (1977)[6]	In situ	Current *v* never or past	1.4
Wright et al (1978)[9]	Invasive	1-14 *v* never or past	1.2
		15+ *v* never or past	3.4
	In situ	1-14 *v* never or past	2.0
		15+ *v* never or past	3.3
	Dysplasia	1-14 *v* never or past	1.0
		15+ *v* never or past	2.3
Harris et al (1980)[10]	In situ	1-14 *v* never or past	2.0
		15+ *v* never or past	3.7
	Severe dysplasia	1-14+ *v* never or past	2.7
		15+ *v* never or past	3.8
	Mild dysplasia	1-14 *v* never or past	3.1
		15+ *v* never or past	3.6
Stellman et al 1980)[11]	CaCx	1-10 *v* never or past	0.7†
		21+ *v* never or past	1.2†

†Estimated from graph

Similarly, Harris et al[10] observed an effect of smoking that persisted after the data were adjusted for contraception and sexual factors and noted that further study was necessary to establish causation.

The study of Stellman et al[11] was the only one to find a relative risk below 1.0 for low levels of smoking. Although heavy smokers were at somewhat increased risk in this study, the authors concluded that their results "are not consistent with a causal hypothesis." Following this publication, an exchange of letters between Winkelstein and Levin[12] and Stellman et al[13] debated the interpretation of these results. Winkelstein and Levin doubted that hospitalized cervical cancer patients were representative and questioned the appropriateness of hospitalized controls as well as the analytic methods used. The authors defended their methods and referred to the fact that prior research had not identified smoking as a risk factor for cervical cancer.

During the following 5 years, extensive research effort was expended in an attempt to clarify this issue. In 1981 Stellman could point to a lack of supporting epidemiologic evidence, but by 1985 ten additional studies had been published, each lending support to the causal hypothesis (Table 29-2).[14-23] Although these studies differ considerably in the populations studied, including an all-black population studied by Trevathan et al,[17] a Mormon population by Lyon et al,[20] and a South African population by Martin and Hill,[21] the results do not appear to vary appreciably with ethnicity. This is in contrast to the finding of Stellman et al,[11] that "the associations found in our data...were opposite in whites and blacks."

With the exception of the study of Greenberg et al,[23] who used the cohort of the Oxford Family Planning Association contraceptive study, all these were case-control studies. The case-control design is the most feasible for addressing this issue, in light of the low incidence of the disease and the need for in-depth interviews to obtain detailed sexual, contraceptive, and smoking histories. The methods of control selection varied widely. These methods included the use of neighborhood or population-based controls,[15,18,20,22] hospitalized controls,[16,21] and family planning clinic patients.[17] Hellberg et al[19] identified both cases and controls at maternity clinics.

Various authors have chosen to study different parts of the gradient of cervical intraepithelial neoplasia. For example, Clark et al first studied only invasive cases[15] and later found similar results in dysplasia patients.[22] Other authors studied one or more of these diagnostic categories.

This group of studies is also quite diverse with respect to the risk factors examined. Only four (Table 29-2) adequately controlled for sexual factors, which are probably the most important confounders in this association.[17,19,20,22] Possible confounding by OC use was examined in five of the more recent studies.[17,19,20,22,23] Since sexual activity and OC use are each positively associated with both smoking and cervical cancer, controlling for these factors can be expected to attenuate the observed association. A number of these studies consider the effect of other potential confounders. Most control for age and some measure of socioeconomic status. In addition, alcohol,[21] diet,[22] and religion[20] have been studied. Nevertheless, in each of these studies a significant association has been observed after the data were adjusted by multivariate analysis. In fact, what is remarkable about this group of studies is the consistency of findings, despite the variability in definition of disease, study design, and analytic methods. Every one of these 20 studies

Table 29-2
Studies Designed to Test Smoking-Cervical Cancer Hypothesis

Author(s)	Case Definition (n)	Control for Sex OC SES	Results
Wigle et al (1980)[14]	Invasive(168)	No No No	Invasive Ca: RR increased from 1.2(10+) to 2.7(31+) pack years In situ: RR increased from 2.2 (10+) to 4.0(20+) pack years
Clarke et al (1982)[15]	Invasive(178)	? No Yes	Adjusted RR 2.2; Increased to 2.9 for 2+ packs/d
Marshall et al (1983)[16]	Cervical cancer (513)	No No Yes	Crude RR: 1.6; No dose response over 1 pack/d
Trevathan et al (1983)[17]	In situ(99)	Yes Yes Yes	RR increased with pack-years (in situ 2.3 to 12.7)
	Dysplasia, severe(81)	Yes Yes Yes	RR increased with early exposure
	Mild-mod(194)	Yes Yes Yes	(no increase after 20 years)
Berggren (1983)[18]	Preinvasive(609)	No No No	Crude RR 2.73; RR decreases with age (9.5 to 1.5)
Hellberg	In situ + Dysplasia, severe(72) Moderate(42)	Yes Yes Yes	Crude RR 4.3 (1983) Adjusted RR not stated
Lyon et al (1983)[20]	In situ(217)	Yes Yes Yes	Adjusted RR 4.1 (LDS) Adjusted RR 1.8 (non LDS) RR decreases with age (17.0-1.6)
Martin and Hill (1984)[2]	Cervical cancer (257)	No No No	After adjusting for alcohol, smoking RR 1.3
Clark et al	Dysplasia(250)	Yes Yes Yes	Current *v* never (1985) Controlling for OC: RR 3.1 Controlling for SES, OC and sex RR 1.9
Greenberg et al (1985)[22]	Invasive(17) In situ(84) Dysplasia(94)	No Yes Yes	Overall trend with dose Adjusted RR (15+ *v* never): Invasive 3.5 In situ 1.8 Dysplasia 2.2

OC = oral contraceptive, SES = socioeconomic status, RR = relative risk.

finds an increased relative risk associated with smoking, which is not explained by any of the risk factors considered.

BIOLOGICAL GRADIENTS

This body of literature suggests a number of biological gradients that tend to support a causal interpretation of these data. First, a dose response has been observed in every instance but one[16] whenever exposure has been quantified. This is true whether smoking is quantified by intensity (packs/day), duration, or both (pack-years) (Figure 29-1).[17]

Second, there appears to be a gradient of risk with increasing severity of disease (Table 29-3). In five studies relative risk estimates are presented for more than one disease category.[9,10,17,22,23] In all but one of these,[10] the relative risk estimates are positively related to severity of disease.

Several studies have found relative risk to decrease with increasing age.[17,18,20] In addition, the effect of age at which a woman starts smoking was carefully examined by Trevathan et al,[17] who found that risk is highest among women who begin to smoke as teen-agers. This trend is seen after total pack-years of smoking is controlled for (Figure 29-2). These data suggest that the adolescent cervix is particularly vulnerable to exposure to cigarette smoke, a reasonable hypothesis given the rapid squamous metaplasia occurring at that time. This observation is consistent with the added risk for cervi-

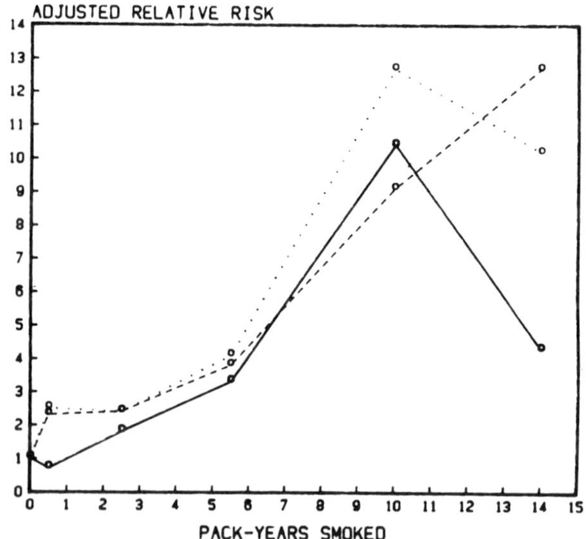

Figure 29-1 Relative risk of cervical intraepithelial neoplasia (CIN) by pack-years of smoking. Dashed line = carcinoma in situ, dotted line = severe dysplasia, solid line = mild to moderate dysplasia.

Table 29-3
Relative Risk for Smoking by Severity of Disease

Author	Dysplasia Mild-Moderate	Severe	All	In Situ	Invasive
Wright et al (1978)[9]			2.3	3.3	3.4
Harris et al (1980)[10]	3.7	3.7		3.1	
Trevathan et al (1983)[17]	2.6	3.0		4.2	
Clark et al (1985)[22]			1.9		2.2
Greenberg et al (1985)[23]		1.8	1.9	1.9	3.0

cal cancer associated with early age at first coitus. The young women at greatest risk may be those exposed simultaneously to early smoking, early sexual activity, and OC use, although no data are yet available to confirm this.

LABORATORY RESULTS SUPPORTING A CAUSAL INTERPRETATION

Recently, Sasson et al[24] measured the levels of nicotine and cotinine in the cervical fluids of smokers and nonsmokers. They found that levels of

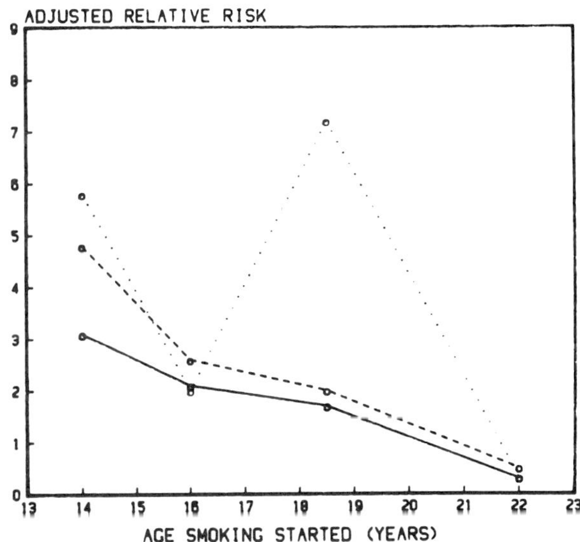

Figure 29-2 Relative risk of CIN by age smoking started. See legend to Figure 29-1.

these primary and secondary smoke constituents were 100 to 200 times higher in smokers than in nonsmokers. Furthermore, although the cotinine levels in serum and cervical fluid were similar, the nicotine levels were between ten and 10,000 times higher in the cervical fluid of smokers. Clearly smoke constituents can and do accumulate in the cervical mucus.

Holly et al[25] conducted a pilot study to determine the mutagenicity of cervical mucus and whether the response to the Ames/Salmonella microsomal test is related to a woman's smoking status. They demonstrated that the relative risk estimate for a positive test result was 4.7 for current smokers compared with nonsmokers. Only women who had smoked within eight hours of sample collection were positive.

CONCLUSION

The large, consistent body of data outlined above is unlikely to be the result of chance. Therefore, the observed association is either an artifact arising from some unmeasured confounding factor or it is causal. Winkelstein et al[26] have shown that any such "mystery confounder" must be strongly related to both smoking and cervical cancer. For example, if the odds ratio for smoking and lung cancer is 2.5, the measure of association between this unknown confounder and both smoking and disease must be approximately 5.0 or more (Appendix A). Moreover, this relationship must hold at each level of exposure, and the unknown confounder must demonstrate the same biological gradients with both smoking and disease as have been observed between smoking and cervical cancer. Thus it is highly unlikely, though not impossible, that such a strong risk factor for disease would remain unknown after the extensive study to which cervical cancer has been subjected.

More likely, the relationship between smoking and cervical neoplasia is a causal one. However, we do not yet understand the relationship of this factor to other known risk factors, particularly infectious agents. MacDonald[27] has suggested that smoking may lead to a compromised immune system, which in turn might increase the risk of cervical cancer among women exposed to an infectious agent. In support of this hypothesis the author cites Ferson et al[28] who reported reduced "natural killing" capacity of blood leukocytes among male smokers compared with nonsmoking controls. Although the mechanism of action remains uncertain, the body of evidence is convincing and supports the conclusion of Austin,[29] that "we can now add cervical cancer to the list of tobacco-caused diseases."

REFERENCES

1. Naguib SM, Lunden FE, Davis HJ: Relation of various epidemiologic factors to cervical cancer as determined by a screening program. *Obstet Gynecol* 1966;28:451-459.

Appendix A
The Mystery Confounder (M)

1 Without controlling for M

OR_{SD} = 2.5

	Case	Control	Total
Smoker	75	55	130
Nonsmoker	25	45	70
	100	100	200

2 Controlling for M

Strata 1
Low level of M
OR_{SD1} = 1.3

	Case	Control	Total
Smoker	15	30	45
Nonsmoker	15	40	55
	30	70	100

Strata 2
High level of M
OR_{SD2} = 1.2

	Case	Control	Total
Smoker	60	25	85
Nonsmoker	10	5	15
	70	30	100

3 How strongly is M associated with disease?

OR_{MD} = 5.4

	Case	Control	Total
High M	70	30	100
Low M	30	70	100
	100	100	200

4 How strongly is M associated with smoking?

OR_{MS} = 6.9

	Smoker	Nonsmoker	Total
High M	85	15	100
Low M	45	55	100
	130	70	200

2. Thomas DB: An epidemiologic study of carcinoma in situ and squamous dysplasia of the uterine cervix. *Am J Epidemiol* 1973;98:10-28.
3. Kessler II, Kulcar Z, Zimolo A, et al: Cervical cancer in Yugoslavia. II. Epidemiologic factors of possible etiologic significance. *J Natl Cancer Inst* 1974;53:51-60.
4. Cederlof R, Friberg L, Hrubec Z, et al: *The Relationship of Smoking and Some Social Covariables to Mortality and Cancer Morbidity. A Ten Year Follow-up in a Probability Sample of 55,000 Swedish Subjects Age 18 to 69.* Stockholm, Department of Environmental Hygiene, Karolinska Institute, 1975.
5. Hirayama T: Prospective studies on cancer epidemiology based on a census population in Japan, in Bucolossi P, Veronesi U, Casinelli N (eds): *Proceedings of Eleventh International Cancer Congress,* Florence, 1974. Amsterdam, Excerpta Medica, 1975, vol 3, pp 26-35.
6. Peritz E, Ramcharan S, Frank J, et al: The incidence of cervical cancer and duration of oral contraceptive use. *Am J Epidemiol* 1977;106:462-469.
7. Williams RR, Horm JW: Association of cancer sites with tobacco and alcohol consumption and socioeconomic status of patients: interview study from the Third National Cancer Survey. *J Natl Cancer Inst* 1977;58:525-547.
8. Winkelstein W: Smoking and cancer of the uterine cervix: hypothesis. *Am J Epidemiol* 1977;106:257-259.
9. Wright H, Vessey MP, Kenward B, et al: Neoplasia and dysplasia of the cervix uteri and contraception: a possible protective effect of the diaphragm. *Br J Cancer* 1978;38:273-279.
10. Harris RWC, Brinton LA, Cowdell RH, et al: Characteristics of women with dysplasia or carcinoma in situ of the cervix uteri. *Br J Cancer* 1980;42:359-369.
11. Stellman SD, Austin H, Wynder EL: Cervix cancer and cigarette smoking: A case-control study. *Am J Epidemiol* 1980;111:383-388.
12. Winkelstein W, Levin L: Confounded confounding. *Am J Epidemiol* 1981;113:99-101.
13. Stellman SD, Austin H, Winder EL: The authors reply. *Am J Epidemiol* 1981;113:101-103.
14. Wigle DT, Mao Y, Grace M: Re: Smoking and cancer of the uterine cervix: hypothesis. *Am J Epidemiol* 1980;111:125127.
15. Clarke EA, Morgan RW, Newman AM: Smoking as a risk factor in cancer of the cervix: additional evidence from a case-control study. *Am J Epidemiol* 1982;115:59-66.
16. Marshall JR, Graham S, Byers T, et al: Diet and smoking in the epidemiology of cancer of the cervix. *J Natl Cancer* Inst 1983;70:847-851.
17. Trevathan E, Layde P, Webster LA, et al: Cigarette smoking and dysplasia and carcinoma in situ of the uterine cervix. *JAMA* 1983;250:499-502.
18. Berggren G, Sjostedt S: Preinvasive carcinoma of the cervix uteri and smoking. *Acta Obstet Gynecol Scand* 1983;62:593-598.
19. Hellberg D, Valentin J, Nilsson S: Smoking as risk factor in cervical neoplasia. *Lancet* 1983;8365:1497.
20. Lyon JL, Gardner JW, West DW, et al: Smoking and carcinoma in situ of the uterine cervix. *Am J Public Health* 1983;73:558-562.
21. Martin P, Hill GB: Cervical cancer in relation to tobacco and alcohol consumption in Lesotho, Southern Africa. *Cancer Detect Prev* 1984;7:109-115.

22. Clark EA, Hatcher J, McKeown-Evssen GE, et al: Cervical dysplasia: Association with sexual behavior, smoking and oral contraceptive use? *Am J Obstet Gynecol* 1985;151:612-616.
23. Greenberg ER, Vessey M, McPherson K, et al: Cigarette smoking and cancer of the uterine cervix. *Br J Cancer* 1985;51:139-141.
24. Sasson IM, Haley NJ, Hoffman D, et al: Cigarette smoking and neoplasia of the uterine cervix: smoke constituents in cervical mucus. *N Engl J Med* 1985;312:315-316.
25. Holly EA, Petrakis NL, Friend NF, et al: Mutagenic cervical mucus in women smokers, abstracted. *Am J Epidemiol* 1985;122:518.
26. Winkelstein W, Shillitoe EJ, Brand R, et al: Further comments on cancer of the uterine cervix, smoking and herpesvirus infection. *Am J Epidmiol* 1984;114:1-8.
27. MacDonald HN: Smoking and oral contraception in cancer of the cervix. *Lancet* 1982;2:989.
28. Ferson M, Edwards A, Lind A, et al: Low natural killer-cell activity and immunoglobulin levels associated with smoking in human subjects. *Int J Cancer* 1979;23:603-609.
29. Austin DF: Smoking and cervical cancer, editorial. *JAMA* 1983;250:516-517.

30 *Research Issues in Smoking and Cervical Neoplasia*

Gary S. Grubb

Cervical neoplasia is the only gynecologic cancer that is positively associated with smoking. Although in several studies a clear relationship has been shown between smoking and cervical neoplasia,[1-4] understanding of this relationship has not developed substantially in the last 5 years. Because cervical neoplasia is known to be a sexually transmitted disease, researchers in the field are instead trying to find the "etiologic agent" for this cancer. However, the potential agent receiving the most attention, human *Papillomavirus*, usually requires an associated carcinogenic agent for malignant transformation in tumor models.[5] Therefore, many researchers have suggested that smoking could play an integral role in the etiology of cervical neoplasia. Further research on smoking could give direction and needed support to investigations of sexually transmitted etiologic agents.

A second possible reason for the slow development of this field of research is that the commonly accepted mechanisms for smoking effects, that is, direct contact (eg, in the oral cavity and lungs) or concentration during excretion (eg, in the kidney and bladder) could not account for a relationship of smoking with cervical neoplasia. Sasson et al at the American Health Foundation[6] demonstrated a potential carcinogenic mechanism through the concentration of nicotine in cervical mucus. This concentration is probably due to pH-trapping of the basic smoking constituents in the acidic vaginal environment. There may also be a selective sequestering of certain other smoking constituent compounds in the mucus. The mechanism appears to have a high interindividual variation, since the ratio of the nicotine concentration in cervical mucus to that in serum may vary more than ten-fold. We do not know what accounts for this variation, yet it may determine which smokers are more likely to develop cervical neoplasia.

Despite the slow pace of research, the field has much potential for advancement. Research can follow three lines of investigation: the role of cervical mucus, the dose-response association between smoking and cervical neoplasia, and the biologic mechanism of smoking's effects on the cervix.

First, it will be important to delineate the role of cervical mucus. How do variations in the physical and chemical properties of cervical mucus, induced by changes in the menstrual cycle, oral contraceptive use, and aging, affect the absorption of nicotine into the mucus? Perhaps these changes account for the wide variation in the ratios of nicotine concentration in serum to that in cervical mucus. In addition, nicotine levels in cervical mucus must be correlated with those in the cervical stroma or local circulation. That is, how effectively does nicotine in the cervical mucus penetrate to the basal layers in which neoplastic cells originate?

To evaluate nicotine's potential as an initiator of malignant transformation in the cervix, it will also be useful to know how nicotine levels correlate with the mutagenicity of the cervical mucus, as reported by Holly et al.[7] Other smoking-related carcinogens may concentrate in the cervical mucus and could also act as cocarcinogens. It would help to understand the pharmacokinetics of nicotine and other potential carcinogens in the cervical mucus. Areas of investigation for these compounds include the peak and trough concentrations after smoking, half-life, and bioavailability.

The principal focus of epidemiologic research should be a refined examination of the dose-response relationship between smoking and cervical neoplasia. Current smokers appear to have a higher risk than past smokers; however, this distinction may mask the influence of past smoking, since current smokers may well have smoked more heavily in the past than those who quit. Therefore, more detailed histories of cigarette consumption are needed. These histories should be related to the times when women experienced other major risks for developing cervical neoplasia, that is, at initial sexual intercourse or at exposure to sexually transmitted diseases or contact with multiple sexual partners. The necessity of age-specific data for cigarette consumption means that pack-years is not an adequate measure of exposure.

The biochemical measures of smoking exposure, which can only reflect current and recent exposures, will be useful in cross-sectional and prospective studies. Case-control studies and prospective studies based on exposure data collected in the past must continue to rely on smoking histories. Validation studies of ages of reported smoking, reported cigarette consumption, and brands smoked will help define the level of confidence we can have in detailed, age-specific smoking histories.

To make these smoking histories complete, it will be necessary to assess passive smoking. Passive exposure to smoke will be difficult to measure, not only because of the much lower levels of exposure than those of active smokers, but also because the level and composition of ambient smoke and exposure to smoking constituents are more complicated to measure than simply assessing the cigarette consumption of others in the home or workplace.[8] In addition, problems in recall will have to be dealt with, since it is usually the nonsmoker, not the smoker, who is recalling the amount smoked and when.

A third focus of future research is the mechanism of smoking's association with cervical neoplasia. Potential mechanisms include a direct carcinogenic effect, local vasoconstriction, local immunosuppression, endocrine alterations, and potentiation of oncogenic viral infections. The direct carcinogenic effects of smoking-related compounds that concentrate in the cervix can be examined by in vitro transformation assays.[9] It may be possible to perform these assays with cell lines derived from the squamous metaplasia cells of the cervical transformation zone—the cells that undergo transformation in cervical neoplasia.

When nicotine, a peripheral vasoconstrictor, is concentrated in the cervix, it may significantly compromise the vascular supply to the cervical epithelium, which may inhibit local immunosurveillance. Selective antibody-linked staining of histologic sections can be used to describe the local immunologic activity. Local vasoconstriction may also create local nutritional deficiencies, specifically, deficiencies of vitamins A, C, and E. These vitamins are antioxidants, which may prevent malignant transformation by inactivating free radicals.[10] Radioimmunoassays can quantify the micronutrient levels in tissue samples.

Among premenopausal women, urinary levels of endogenous estrogens are lower in smokers than nonsmokers. Smoking has antiestrogenic effects, which may decrease the risk of endometrial cancer.[11] With regard to cervical cancer and endocrine alterations, oral contraceptive use for 5 or more years appears to be associated with a 1.5- to two-fold increased risk of cervical cancer.[12,13] This suggests that long-term exposure to combined progestogen and estrogen increases the risk of cervical neoplasia. Smoking may well mediate this risk in some way.

A likely mechanism for smoking's effect is the potentiation of oncogenic viral infections of the cervix. Research on cervical neoplasia is now centered on the human *Papillomavirus* (HPV). Five of the more than 30 reported HPV subtypes cause genital warts, and two or three of these subtypes, which are found in less than 10% of genital warts, are associated with a much higher risk of developing cervical neoplasia than the more common HPV subtypes that cause genital warts.[14]

Other HPV subtypes cause condylomas or warts on other parts of the body, such as the skin and larynx; these warts are known to have a high risk of malignant transformation. For this transformation to occur, however, a cocarcinogen appears necessary.[5] In animal tumor models this is often a chemical cocarcinogen. Human *Papillomavirus* is hypothesized to promote malignant transformation, and the cocarcinogen would initiate this process. For example, cattle with intestinal papillomas develop intestinal carcinomas if they eat bracken fern, which contains the carcinogen, quercin. Rabbits with a certain skin papilloma develop skin cancers if the papillomas are coated with polycyclic hydrocarbons. Cigarette smoke contains several substances that could act as a cocarcinogen of HPV. These potential cocarcinogens can be evaluated for their interactive effects with HPV in transformation assays.

Interactive effects between cervical HPV infection and smoking need to be assessed in epidemiologic studies. The dose-response effect of smoking with synergistic carcinogens has been found to be a multiplicative interaction.[15] However, rather than stating whether synergy is or is not present according to statistical criteria, a presentation of the actual risks for the groups exposed to the potentially interacting factors would be useful. Such group-specific data are also useful when a potential cocarcinogen has only marginal interaction and is a confounder for an association between HPV infection and cervical intra-epithelial neoplasia (CIN). In such a case, the evidence for the potential cocarcinogen's interactive effects could be important to understanding its role in the development of CIN. An estimate of risk adjusted for the confounding factor would be less informative. As a model for assessing the relationship between smoking and HPV, the possibility of a multiplicative interaction between smoking and herpes simplex virus type 2 infection was examined in a recent epidemiologic study,[4] but no evidence for an interaction was found. If HPV does play a significant part in causing cervical cancer, it

REFERENCES

1. Trevanthan E, Layde PM, Webster LA, et al: Cigarette smoking and dysplasia and carcinoma in situ of the uterine cervix. *JAMA* 1983;250:499-502.
2. Lyon JL, Gardner JW, West DW, et al: Smoking and carcinoma in situ of the uterine cervix. *Am J Public Health* 1983;73:558-562.

3. Clarke EA, Hatcher J, McKeown-Eyssen GE, et al: Cervical dysplasia: Association with sexual behavior, smoking and oral contraceptive use? *Am J Obstet Gynecol* 1985;151:612-616.
4. Mayberry RM: Cigarette smoking, herpes simplex virus type 2 infection, and cervical abnormalities. *Am J Public Health* 1985;75:676-678.
5. zur Hausen H: Human genital cancer: synergism between two virus infections or synergism between a virus infection and initiating events. *Lancet* 1982;2:1370-1372.
6. Sasson IM, Haley NJ, Hoffman D, et al: Cigarette smoking and neoplasia of the uterine cervix. smoking constituents in cervical mucus. *N Engl J Med* 1985;312:315-316.
7. Holly EA, Petrakis NL, Friend NF, et al: Mutagenic cervical mucus in women smokers. Presented at Society for Epidemiology Research, Chapel Hill, NC, June 19, 1985.
8. US Dept of Health and Human Services: *The Health Consequences of Smoking—Chronic Obstructive Lung Disease: a Report of the Surgeon General.* US Dept of Health and Human Services publication No. (PHS) 480-1440-85-13, Government Printing Office, 1984, pp 366-384.
9. Yee C, Krishnan-Hewlett I, Baker CC, et al: Presence and expression of human *Papillomavirus* sequences in human cervical cell lines. *Am J Pathol* 1985;119:361-366.
10. Romney SL, Palan PR, Duttagupta C, et al: Retinoids and the prevention of cervical dysplasia. *Am J Obstet Gynecol* 1981;141:890-894.
11. Lesko SM, Rosenberg L, Kaufman DW, et al: Cigarette smoking and the risk of endometrial cancer. N Engl J Med 1985;313:593-596.
12. WHO Collaborative Study of Neoplasia and Steroid Contraceptives: Breast cancer, cervical cancer, and depomedroxyprogesterone acetate. *Lancet* 1984;2:1207-1208.
13. Vessey MP, Lawless M, McPherson K, et al: Neoplasia of the cervix uteri and contraception: a possible adverse effect of the pill. *Lancet* 1983;2:930-935.
14. Syrjanen KJ: Current concepts of human *Papillomavirus* infections in the genital tract and their relationship to intraepithelial neoplasia and squamous cell carcinoma. *Obstet Gynecol Surv* 1984;39:252-265.
15. Reif AE: Synergism in carcinogenesis. *J Natl Cancer Inst* 1984;73:25-39.

31 *Smoking and Cancer: Methodologic Considerations*

James E. Higgins

Cigarette smoke originates primarily from two sources: mainstream and sidestream. Mainstream smoke is drawn through the cigarette, which filters some of the active constituents, and is inhaled by the smoker. Sidestream smoke is released from the burning end of the cigarette between puffs. Sidestream smoke contains the same constituents as mainstream smoke, but the concentrations of some, including several known carcinogens, differ. For example, dimethylnitrosamine is 52 times as concentrated in mainstream smoke, methylnaphthalene is 28 times as concentrated, naphthalene is 16 times as concentrated, toluene is five times as concentrated, and benzo(a)pyrene is three times as concentrated.[1,2]

Active smokers are exposed to both mainstream and sidestream smoke. The mainstream smoke is inhaled directly into the lungs and is diluted only by the air taken in with the puff.Passive smokers are primarily exposed to sidestream smoke, which is usually diluted by a much larger volume of air. Approximately 85% of the cigarette smoke in a room is sidestream smoke. The remaining 15% is a combination of exhaled smoke, smoke diffused through the paper wrapping, and smoke from the nonburning end of the cigarette.[1,2]

The number of cigarettes smoked is a good measure of both mainstream and sidestream smoke exposure of active smokers, although the exposure varies with what is smoked and how it is smoked. The exposure of passive smokers is more difficult to quantify. Important factors in determining passive smoke exposure are the type and number of cigarettes smoked and the size and ventilation rate in the room.

MEASURING EXPOSURE

Questionnaires

The most popular method of measuring active and passive smoking is self-reporting by questionnaire. Self-reports are generally inexpensive and easy to collect. There is evidence that smokers underreport consumption,[3] but little is known about the relationship between the level of underreporting and the amount actually smoked. Retrospective estimates of smoking display a strong bias in that approximately 70% of smokers report the number of cigarettes smoked in a day in units of ten.[4]

The most important parameter of exposure is the smoking rate, expressed as a function of age or reproductive history. A questionnaire reconstruction of the smoking rate requires data on the age of initiation, periods of cessation (circumstances of cessation are useful also), dates of reproductive events, and the average daily consumption during each of the active smoking periods. Validation studies of questionnaire-determined smoking rates are needed. Prospective studies and use of medical or insurance records are two possibilities for validation. Additional parameters of smoking that are frequently collected include type(s) of cigarettes smoked, techniques of smoking, other products smoked, and use of smokeless tobacco.

Most often, information on sidestream smoke exposure is obtained by proxy. Reports by next-of-kin on smoking habits of subjects in a cohort study showed a 90% agreement on a crude classification of smoking status (regular, occasional, or never).[5] Agreement on the number of packs smoked per day was 75%, and men were less likely than women to agree with the subject's report. Informants tended to report heavier smoking than the smoker on whom they reported.

Whether an informant who smokes provides more accurate information than a nonsmoker has not been reported. Information on sidestream smoke should include exposure during childhood, from partners, and at the workplace.[6] Simulation indicates that exposure to sidestream smoke at the workplace is four times that received at home.[7]

Biochemical Measures

Biochemical measures, which have been recommended as a more objective alternative to questionnaires,[4] measure constituents of tobacco smoke in blood, urine, saliva, and expired air. The constituents most often measured are carbon monoxide, thiocyanate, and nicotine and/or cotinine. Carbon monoxide is measured in expired air, but the interpretation of levels due to cigarette smoke is confounded by ambient concentrations. For a smoker to be identified accurately, he or she must have smoked in the previous nine hours.

Thiocyanate, a product of cyanide detoxification, accumulates in body fluids and provides an estimate of exposure to hydrogen cyanide in tobacco smoke.[8] Its biological half-life in serum is ten to 14 days. Concentrations are affected by consumption of cabbage, cauliflower, broccoli, beer, and certain beans. Thiocyanate levels are best measured in saliva or serum, but urine is also used.

Nicotine is unique to tobacco, but its half life in serum is only 20 to 60 minutes. Because its metabolite, cotinine, has a 30-hour half-life, cotinine is recommended as a measure of tobacco exposure.

Two locations in the United States that provide laboratory services to analyze blood, urine, and saliva samples for nicotine/cotinine and thiocyanate are:

Naylor Dana Institute for Disease Prevention
American Health Foundation
Valhalla, NY 10595

Division of Epidemiology
School of Public Health
University of Minnesota
611 Beacon Street SE
Minneapolis, MN 55455.

Use of Biochemical Measures

Biochemical measures have been used in several studies of current smoking, especially prevalence studies and studies of smoking cessations.[9,10] Biochemical measures have also been suggested for use in prospective epidemiologic studies. Their value in retrospective studies appears to be limited to improved accuracy of smoking histories reported by adolescents who, in one study, were more likely to report that they smoked if they were informed that they would be given an objective smoking test.[11]

The usefulness of biochemical measures to distinguish between light smokers and nonsmokers has been questioned[12]; however, this may not be a shortcoming, since interest usually focuses on measuring exposure to smoke, whether mainstream or sidestream. Biochemical measures have also been used to estimate smoke exposure of nonsmokers in cigarette equivalents. Among employees at a hospital, nonsmokers were exposed to the equivalent of one to three cigarettes in a four-hour period (nicotine in urine and saliva).[13]

Blood nicotine concentrations in nonsmoking flight attendants, after a 12-hour flight, were estimated to be equivalent to smoking one cigarette.[14] Nonsmoking patrons of a pub, after 2 hours of exposure, were found to have concentrations of carbon monoxide and cotinine equivalent to smoking less than a third of a cigarette.[15] Urinary cotinine was used to determine that a nonsmoker living with a two-pack-a-day smoker is exposed to the equivalent of three cigarettes per day.[16]

SIDESTREAM SMOKE AND REPRODUCTIVE CANCERS

The effect of exposure to sidestream smoke has been reported in four case-control studies of cervical cancer. Buckley et al[17] compared the behavior of the husbands of 31 women with cervical dysplasia, carcinoma in situ, or invasive carcinoma of the cervix with the behavior of husbands of 62 hospital controls. The wives ranged in age from 30 to 70, with an average of 48 years. After the data were adjusted for the number of the husbands' sexual partners (but not for the wives' smoking), women who smoked were at 1.8 times the risk of one of the three conditions studied ($P > .05$).

Hellberg et al compared 132 pregnant women with cervical neoplasia with 260 pregnant controls.[18] The average age of the women was 26 years. Without adjusting the data, the investigators found that women married to smokers were at twice the risk of cervical neoplasia ($P < .01$). The odds ratio, after the data were adjusted for the wives' smoking, was reported to be less than 2.0 and "nonsignificant," but no values were given.

Brown et al investigated 22 cases of carcinoma in situ and 11 cases of invasive carcinoma of the cervix, compared with 27 controls.[19] The ages of the women were not given. A smoking husband was reported to be the most important risk factor, with an unadjusted odds ratio of 3.8. Neither sexual activity nor the women's smoking history were adjusted for.

Sandler et al studied the relationship between passive smoking in adulthood and cancer risk to both men and women.[20] Only exposure to a husband's or wife's smoking was considered. Over 80% of the cases and controls had been married. Included in the malignancies investigated were 101 cases of cervical cancer. After adjustment for age and education of the women, wives with smoking husbands were at 1.8 times the risk of cervical cancer (95% confidence interval, 1.1-3.2). When cervical cancer cases were restricted to nonsmoking women and compared with nonsmoking controls, women with smoking husbands were at 2.1 times the risk (95% confidence interval, 1.2-3.9).

Evidence that passive smoking may be associated with cervical cancer is accumulating. Since exposure measured in cigarette equivalents is less than three cigarettes per day for passive smokers, the strength of the effect in two of the studies[19,20] is puzzling. Perhaps cigarette equivalents is not a valid measure of passive smoking. The evidence linking passive smoking and cervical cancer is not yet convincing but is compelling enough to encourage investigators to measure passive smoking in future studies.

REFERENCES

1. US Dept of Health, Education, and Welfare: *Smoking and Health: A Report of the Surgeon General.* US Dept of Health and Human Services publication No. (PHS) 79-50066, 1979.
2. US Dept of Health and Human Services: *The Health Consequences of Smoking--Cancer: A Report of the Surgeon General.* US Dept of Health and Human Services publication No. (PHS) 82-50179, 1982.
3. Warner K: Possible increases in the underreporting of cigarette consumption. *J Am Stat Assoc* 1978;73:314-318.

4. Pechacek TF, Fox BH, Murray DM, et al: Review of techniques for measurement of smoking behavior, in Matarazzo JD, Weiss SM, Herd JA, Miller NE, Weiss SM (eds): *Behavioral Health: A Handbook of Health Enhancement and Disease Prevention.* New York, Wiley, 1984, pp 729-754.
5. Rogot E, Reid DD: The validity of data from next of kin in studies of mortality among migrants. *Int J Epidemiol* 1975;4:51-53.
6. Repace JL, Lowrey AH: Modeling exposure of nonsmokers to ambient tobacco smoke. Presented at Seventy-Sixth Annual Meeting of the Air Pollution Control Association, Atlanta, June 19-24, 1983.
7. Sandler DP, Everson RB, Wilcox AJ, et al: Cancer risk in adulthood from early life exposure to parent's smoking. *Am J Public Health* 1985;75:487-492.
8. Vessey C: Thiocyanates and cigarette consumption, in Greenlaugh RM (ed): *Smoking and Arterial Disease.* London, Pitman Press, 1981.
9. Williams CL, Eng A, Botvin GJ, et al: Validation of student's self-reported cigarette smoking status with plasma cotinine levels. *Am J Public Health* 1979;69:1272-1274.
10. Bliss RE, O'Connell KA: Problems with thiocyanate as an index of smoking status: a critical review with suggestions for improving the usefulness of biochemical measures in smoking cessation research. *Health Psychol* 1984;3:563-581.
11. Bauman KE, Dent CW: Influence of an objective measure on self-reports of behavior. *J Appl Psychol* 1982;67;623-628.
12. Petitti DB, Friedman GD, Kahn W: Accuracy of information on smoking habits provided on self-administered research questionnaires. *Am J Public Health* 1981;71:308-3ll.
13. Feyerabend C, Higenbottam T, Russell MAH: Nicotine concentrations in urine and saliva of smokers and non-smokers. *Br Med J* 1982;284:1002-1004.
14. Foliart D, Benowitz NL, Becker CE: Passive absorption of nicotine in airline flight attendants, letter to the editor. *N Engl J Med* 1983;308:1105.
15. Jarvis MJ, Russell MAH, Feyerabend C: Absorption of nicotine and carbon monoxide from passive smoking under natural conditions of exposure. *Thorax* 1983;38:829-833.
16. Matsukura S, Taminato T, Norikazu K, et al: Effects of environmental smoke on urinary cotinine excretion in nonsmokers. *N Engl J Med* 1984;311:828-832.
17. Buckley JD, Doll R, Harris RWC, et al: Case-control study of the husbands of women with dysplasia or carcinoma of the cervix uteri. *Lancet* 1981;2:1010-1014.
18. Hellberg D, Valentin J, Nilsson S: Smoking as risk factor in cervical neoplasia. *Lancet* 1983;2:1497.
19. Brown DC, Pereira L, Garner JB: Cancer of the cervix and the smoking husband. *Can Family Physician* 1982;28:499-502.
20. Sandler DP, Everson RP, Wilcox AJ: Passive smoking in adulthood and cancer risk. *Am J Epidemiol* 1985;121:37-48.

32 *Public Health and Public Policy Issues*

John Pinney

Prior to the release of the 1979 Surgeon General's Report on the Health Consequences of Smoking, the effects of smoking on women had received little national attention. Many people, public health officials included, had assumed that since women had not manifested the same high levels of smoking-related morbidity and mortality as men, they were somehow protected from or less susceptible to the cardiovascular, respiratory and cancer risks demonstrated for male smokers.

The 1979 Report captured the attention of health officials and the public by establishing once and for all the unshakable scientific validity of the case against smoking. It also set the stage for new emphasis on women and smoking by concluding, "Women who smoke like men die like men who smoke."[1] And it brought together for the first time the extensive and frightening evidence on the effects of maternal smoking on fetal and infant health.

The following year's Surgeon General's Report was devoted entirely to the problem of women and smoking in an effort to redress the imbalance of attention and concern and to elicit new public health and public policy discussions about remedies. Policy makers at the federal level hoped that the evidence about the special health risks of women smokers and the outright targeting of the women's market by the cigarette manufacturers would motivate the women's health movement to address the smoking issue. Raising the level of concern among health care providers about the health consequences shared by male and female smokers was an equally important goal, reflected in public information campaigns with themes such as "Lung cancer is an equal opportunity tragedy."[2]

The tragedy of the increasing death rate from lung cancer in women was the most enduring message to emanate from this period. The image of lung cancer surpassing breast cancer as the leading cause of cancer death among women was and is a powerful message that can be graphically depicted and tracked as it becomes a reality. The impact of smoking on reproductive health has not captured the same degree of attention, yet in the broader context of health and public policy, it is an issue of equal or greater significance.

PUBLIC HEALTH SIGNIFICANCE

Although overall, smoking in the United States has declined from 42% of adults in 1964[3] to 30% in 1985[4] smoking among women is not declining as rapidly as it is among men. In fact, the smoking rate among young women aged 20 to 30 years has increased slightly in recent years. This is cause for concern since these women are the role models for the next generation of young women, and since their most fertile years and their smoking will affect not only the outcome of their pregnancies but also the attitudes of their children about smoking. The combined human and economic costs of low birth weight and other effects of smoking such as spontaneous abortion, perinatal mortality, and developmental deficits are unacceptably high.

Compared to women in the United States and other developed countries, women in less developed countries are far less likely to smoke. However, in any setting where the accessibility or quality of health care may be limited, a factor which poses an additional but avoidable risk to pregnancy outcome constitutes a serious public health problem. And while data are not available to assess overall trends in smoking among women in less developed countries, the loss of markets in developed countries has spurred increased marketing efforts which may result in significant increases in smoking among these women. Also, smoking patterns in less developed countries have followed fairly closely those in developed countries—smoking begins among men of higher socioeconomic status and moves down the socioeconomic scale; women lag men by several decades in the uptake of smoking by significant numbers of women. If the latter part of this pattern holds true, smoking among women will surely be a global public health problem.

POLICY IMPLICATIONS

At this point, it is important to look at smoking and reproductive health in the broader context of emerging public policies addressed to smoking. The last decade has seen enormous growth in the extent, power, and effectiveness of public health and political efforts aimed at preventing the spread and reducing the prevalence of smoking. From Africa to Asia to India, in Europe, Scandinavia, North and South America, slow but constant progress has been made in organizing and directing public policy efforts against smoking and the power of the cigarette manufacturers. Much remains to be done, but the experience and confidence gained from successes such as advertising bans in Sudan, workplace restrictions in the United States and growing awareness worldwide of the dangers of smoking have helped create a public policy base that will be of great value to all who are working for the adoption of anti-smoking policies.

The issue of smoking and reproductive health offers an excellent opportunity to formulate policies that discourage smoking while protecting the health of the fetus and the newborn. Even the cigarette manufacturers have found it difficult to assail the evidence on smoking and reproductive health or the basis for encouraging pregnant women to quit. And a large number of women can and do quit while they are pregnant. The challenge is to find ways to help them stay quit after the birth of their child, to help their spouses quit, and to ensure the newborn a smokefree environment and a future in which the odds of taking up smoking are greatly reduced.

Policy options must be developed that deal with the unique problems of smoking and reproductive health. In the United States, restrictions on smoking in the workplace show promise for encouraging smokers to quit and reducing the risk of passive smoke exposure. Special efforts by those same employers to help their pregnant employees to quit smoking would seem reasonable and warranted. Both women and men in general need a better understanding of the full range of risks which their smoking poses for their infants. Cigarette marketing and advertising aimed at women and depicting smoking as socially acceptable, healthy, and attractive can only make such educational efforts more difficult. Activist strategies to limit or ban such advertising are increasingly being considered or launched. Groups concerned about women's health must recognize that smoking is a women's health issue worthy of commitment and action, even to the extent of jeopardizing cigarette advertising revenues by taking stronger editorial positions in women's magazines.

The risks of inaction are obvious—a continuation of the avoidable toll in infant mortality and morbidity associated with smoking; the possible increase in smoking among successive cohorts of women, in the United States and in other countries; the lost opportunity of creating nonsmoking generations of children. Without policies aimed at preventing and reducing smoking among women in their childbearing years, we may see successful efforts by transnational cigarette manufacturers to extend smoking to those women who for sociocultural and religious reasons have not yet taken up smoking.

In the United States, it seems too little attention was paid to women and the special health risks of their smoking until too late—the cigarette companies targeted women and succeeded in creating a true women's market. It is hoped, this lesson will encourage other countries to act now.

REFERENCES

1. US Dept of Health and Human Services: *Smoking and Health: A Report of the Surgeon General.* US Dept of Health, Education, and Welfare, publication No. (PHS) 79-55071, Government Printing Office, 1979.
2. US Dept of Health and Human Services: *The Health Consequences of Smoking for Women: A Report of the Surgeon General.* Government Printing Office, 1980.

3. US Dept of Health and Human Services: *Cancer: A Report of the Surgeon General.* US Dept of Health and Human Services, publication No. (PHS) 82-50179, Government Printing Office, 1982.
4. National Center for Health Statistics: *Provisional data from the Health Promotion and Disease Prevention Supplement to the National Health Interview Survey: US, January-March 1985.* Advanced Data from Vital and Health Statistics, No. 113. US Dept of Health and Human Services publication No. (PHS) 86-1250, Hyattsville, Md, 1985.

33 *Smoking and Women at Work*

Diana Chapman Walsh

As women have entered the workplace in unprecedented and growing numbers, the health issues surrounding fertility, pregnancy, and childbearing have increasingly challenged employers. Meanwhile, rising health care costs, interest in health promotion, and a rapidly changing legal context are compelling employers to formulate policies toward smoking as a public health issue. These two trends, however, are rarely seen as related, and little has been done to address the potential interaction between smoking and reproductive health in the context of work. This paper asks how realistic it is to expect that programs to discourage smoking in the workplace will become an important part of an overall campaign to discourage smoking during pregnancy.

The workplace is viewed as a good setting for addressing the problem of smoking and reproductive health, since it provides access to most adults and offers program designers convenience and the opportunity to mobilize a wide range of vehicles. The workplace makes it possible to establish a policy framework that includes manipulation of the "corporate culture"; use organizational and social supports; create financial incentives for individuals and work groups; mount educational campaigns; and offer a range of clinical interventions and behavioral modification techniques.[1] The occupational setting also allows repeated, extended follow-up to deal with relapses.

As compelling as the logic may be for workplace interventions, a number of problems arise. Policies on smoking, work, and reproductive health are each highly charged, so the combination may be that much more difficult. Successful establishment of programs to reduce smoking in the workplace will require coming to grips with social, legal, and economic issues.

The social context shaping employers' responses to the issues of reproductive health and work includes the increase in number and proportion of women in the work force, in the absence of coherent social policy. Unlike 75 other nations, the United States has no guarantee of paid leave and job protection for pregnancy and childbirth.[2] A 1979 amendment to title VII of the Civil Rights Act of 1964 was an initial step that left many gaps.[3] Known as the Pregnancy Disability Act, this law was intended to prohibit employers from discriminating against pregnant women in any area of employment and benefit programs. It requires employers to treat pregnancy like any other disability but applies only to employers with 15 or more employees that have existing benefit plans. Five states have added statutes mandating more extensive benefits during pregnancy, but these still leave many working women, 85% of whom may become pregnant during their working lives,[2] without coverage. A growing proportion of women who stay on the job while pregnant return to work within a year of giving birth. This proportion would presumably be greater if their jobs were protected. Moreover, the increasing involvement of fathers in early parenting duties makes job flexibility for childbearing attractive to men as well as women.

From a purely economic standpoint, it may be worth an employer's while to attend, however cautiously, to the impact of smoking on reproductive outcome. Maternity-related costs nearly always rank among the top three items in employee benefit packages and (depending on the age and sex structure of the employee and dependent population) often lead the list. This is because uncomplicated delivery is one of the most frequent causes of hospitalization in healthy populations. When complications arise, the costs rapidly multiply. With mounting interest in "high-cost users" of health care[4] and in means of reducing health costs, evaluations of how smoking translates to dollars are inevitable.

The economic argument for employer action rested originally on the work of Kristein,[5] whose estimates have been extended to motivate companies to invest in programs to promote employees' health. The hyperbole that sometimes ensues, however, can undermine the credibility of health promotion. For example, a recent textbook on worksite health promotion calls smoking "the leading cause of absenteeism in industrial worker populations,"[6] a claim that ignores numerous other variables that predict absenteeism.[7] Focusing on a single risk factor, without acknowledging related effects that may explain at least part of the association (drinkers smoke and smokers drink, and both have more than their share of accidents and lost work days), overstates the case for a single health promotion initiative.

Corporate smoking policies have evolved through three generations. The first reflects special circumstances, which include customer relations, equipment conservation, the incompatibility of smoking with work routines, or extreme hazards that react synergistically with smoking.[8] An example is the Johns-Manville policy, which was stimulated by the crisis of asbestos-related disease.[9] A second-generation policy, which still predominates in American industry, involves balancing the demands of smokers and nonsmokers, establishing even-handed and conciliatory policies, and providing cessation programs on a voluntary, episodic basis, usually through outside organizations.[10] A few companies have advanced on the smoking issue to a third-generation approach, generally as part of a comprehensive health promotion program. This approach seeks to change the corporate culture so that a nonsmoking lifestyle is seen as the clear norm. The goal is to move smokers gradually through successive phases of cessation, while providing social support from within the organization, similar to worksite programs to control hypertension.[11] This type of program raises the larger question of whether and how the workplace can serve as an appropriate site for the management of chronic disease.[12] Few companies have progressed this far,[13] but in state and national samples, 30% to 50% of large employers report that they restrict or prohibit smoking in at least some work areas.[14]

A recent example of a third-generation program may be a bellwether for the future of worksite smoking policies because, unlike previous policies, it does not involve a health care or other special-interest firm and may therefore be generalizable to a wide variety of American corporations. Effective in 1985, Pacific Northwest Bell, a 15,000-employee telephone company, banned smoking in all its locations (including a 32-story building). The decision followed over 2 years of deliberation, stimulated by pressure from nonsmoking employees. None of the senior officers of the company are themselves smokers, and the legal department was said to have been concerned about potential liability for harm to nonsmoking employees. The possibility of creating smoking lounges was explored and rejected as prohibitively expensive. Ultimately the decision was made to ban smoking and for a time to underwrite fully the costs of cessation programs for employees and their dependents. The union local elected to take no stand supporting or opposing the management policy, and close observers are predicting that such a policy may in time become commonplace.

Much remains to be learned about how to target smoking cessation efforts to women workers who smoke and how to capitalize on the motivational factors associated with pregnancy. Research on working women is needed if workplace initiatives are to be effective. One barrier is that the number of pregnancies among employees in a single location, even a large one, is generally too small to justify a special program or to support research on alternative strategies.

If smoking policy is to be guided by economic considerations, then public policy will have to reckon with the fact that one payer's cost containment is almost invariably another's new cost burden. Refusing to employ smokers is an effective way for companies to rapidly reduce their smoking-related costs. Unaccompanied by an effective campaign to reduce the absolute numbers of smokers, however, the burden is merely shifted to the smoker, his new employer, or the unemployment system. If costs are the issue, then restrictions limited to the workplace miss spouses and dependent children, who normally account for more than half of health benefit costs. As the desire to moderate costs increasingly draws employers' attention to groups of high-cost users in their employee and dependent populations, the insurance principle is lost to a new kind of discrimination. This makes it even more important that analyses that affect these decisions be sound. They will surely not be if they examine one risk factor at a time, without considering that risk behaviors tend to be intertwined in a complex web that has been referred to as a "risk syndrome."[15]

Setting policy then becomes a problem of where to draw lines. If the goal is to save the costs associated with smoking's health effects, then merely banning smoking on the job is not enough. Smoking has to stop both on and off the job, which is tantamount to saying that employers should be allowed to refuse to hire smokers. If employability can be based on smoking both on and off the job, then what other lifestyle factors could be used to discriminate? So far, denying smokers work has been limited to situations where smoking synergistically increases health risks associated with a particular job, as in the asbestos industry. If more than one factor—in this case, smoking and work—can have a combined adverse effect on reproduction greater than either one by itself, then careful thought needs to be given to the equity issues that may arise.

If policy in the workplace is to reflect predominantly the need for improving health, then the issues of occupational segregation and quality of jobs are raised. Companies where health-oriented programs are best developed are the large corporations in the industrial and financial services sector, where women are underrepresented. That women's jobs are still concentrated in industries notable for their lack of rudimentary health benefits undermines the notion that a workplace strategy to mitigate the harm of smoking on reproduction is destined to have a major national impact.

CONCLUSIONS

Framers of policies on smoking and reproductive health have to consider the two areas of reproductive hazards and smoking, both of which are complex and controversial. It therefore seems unlikely that many employers will aggressively address the specific effects of smoking on reproductive outcome. If the nonsmoking policy of Pacific Northwest Bell becomes widespread, then such a broad policy will help reduce smoking before and during pregnancy. Designing effective and lasting policies relating smoking to work will require employers to view their employees as "human capital" and treat reduction of their health risks as essential to the organization's long-term survival. Rare is the employer who thinks and acts in these terms. The campaign against smoking during pregnancy will therefore most likely be waged outside the workplace.

Acknowledgments

The work on which this article draws has been funded in part by a grant from the Pew Memorial Trust.

REFERENCES

1. Walsh DC: Corporate smoking policies: a review and an analysis. *J Occup Med* 1984;26:17-22.
2. Kamerman SB, Kahn AJ, Kinston P: *Maternity Policies and Working Women.* New York, Columbia University Press, 1983.
3. Walsh DC, Egdahl RH: *Women, Work and Health: Challenges to Corporate Policy.* New York, Springer-Verlag, 1980.
4. Zook C, Moore F: High-cost users of medical care. *N Engl J Med* 1980;302:996-1002.
5. Kristein MM: How much can business expect to profit from smoking cessation? *Prev Med* 1983;12:358-381.
6. Schwartz RM, Rollins PL: Measuring the cost benefit of wellness strategies. *Business and Health* 1985;2(10):24-26.
7. O'Donnell MP, Ainsworth T: *Health Promotion in the Workplace.* New York, John Wiley & Sons, 1984.
8. Bennett D, Levy BS: Smoking policies and smoking cessation programs of large employers in Massachusetts. *Am J Public Health* 1980;70:629-631.
9. Cenci L: *Smoking and the Workplace: A Paper of the National Interagency Council on Smoking and Health.* New York, Academy of Medicine, 1980.
10. Orleans CS, Shipley RH: Worksite smoking cessation initiatives: review and recommendations. *Addict Behav* 1982;7:1-16.
11. Foote A, Erfurt JC: Hypertension control: formula for success. *Business and Health* 1984;2:13-18.
12. Walsh DC: Is there a doctor in-house? *Harvard Bus Rev* 1984;62:84.
13. Shepard DS, Pearlman LA: Healthy habits that pay off. *Business and Health* 1985;2(4):37-41.
14. *Smoking Policies in Large Corporations.* Los Angeles, CA: Human Resources Policy Institute, 1985.
15. Perry CL, Jessor R: The concept of health promotion and the prevention of adolescent drug abuse. *Health Educ Q* 1985; 12(2):pp 169-184.

34 *Smoking Control Policies and Female Smoking Habits in Less Developed Countries*

Mario Rigatto, M.A. Arabi, Husain A. Al-Mumen, Joseph O. M. Pobee

BRAZIL

In Brazil, women's addiction to tobacco must be considered the number one priority as far as the public health issue of tobacco is concerned, for several reasons: one third of the adult female population smokes; the percentage of pregnant women (especially those in the lower socioeconomic groups[1]) who smoke is increasing[2]; smoking prevalence in teen-aged girls recently surpassed that in boys[3]; and oral contraceptives are widely used by women who are unaware of the risks associated with concurrent OC and tobacco use.[4] In 1975 a public antismoking campaign led by physicians, started in Rio Grande do Sul, the southernmost state of Brazil, where 50% of Brazilian tobacco is cultivated. In a few years, this campaign gained national dimensions. The main objectives of the campaign have been, first, to inform and to motivate the population, and second, to stimulate governmental action.

The task was difficult. Brazil is the fourth largest producer of tobacco and one of its larger consumers in the world. From an economic viewpoint, no other country is more dependent on tobacco than Brazil: 10% to 12% of its total federal tax revenue comes from tobacco.[5] We did not rank a war against the tobacco industry as a priority. The tobacco industry is made up of multinational institutions governed entirely by money. The moral behavior of a multinational institution must be determined by the government of the country affected by the institution. No government is expected to allow activities harmful to its people to be developed within the territory under its control.

We quickly found that our government was not ready for action. It neither realized the extent of the problem nor had the necessary political courage to face it. So we concentrated our work on the community as the main force capable of changing governmental attitudes. As a consequence of this approach, several municipal laws prohibiting smoking in public places have been passed. A few state and local laws were also approved, but Brazil has not had a single federal law restricting tobacco.[6] Forty proposals of law, already approved by the Health Committee of our Congress, await a majority vote. The economic forces of the Brazilian government have maintained a firm stand against banning tobacco.

In spite of these difficulties, the results have been encouraging. The steady growth in the annual consumption of cigarettes in Brazil, at a rate of about 7% a year, came to a halt in 1980, when peak sales of 143 billion cigarettes were recorded. Since 1980, cigarette consumption has been steadily declining at a rate of about 3% a year. In 1983 the sales reached 129 billion cigarettes, a 10% decrease from 1980 levels. The importance of this reduction in absolute terms is magnified in relative terms by the vegetative growth of the population—2.5% per year—and by the escalation of the advertising budget of the tobacco industry, which has doubled since 1980.

The experience gained with the antitobacco campaign in Brazil provides the following lessons for similar campaigns in other developing countries:

1. Physicians and other health personnel cannot win the war by themselves, but a strong stand by the medical forces is mandatory. They master the scientific arguments, the only weapons that have proved capable against the tobacco forces. Besides their scientific authority, physicians offer the best example of renouncing profit in favor of the common good. No professional class will lose more money than medical doctors if the tobacco ban succeeds.
2. Next to physicians and health personnel as a whole, the most important allies are teachers, particularly those in the elementary school.
3. The use of the media is too expensive for most antismoking campaigns, but space can be gained by presenting the information as news.
4. More important than counteracting propaganda is disseminating information about the health risks of tobacco. To ensure action, information must be quantitatively adequate and qualitatively adjusted to the target population. For instance, the effective arguments for children are not the same as those for adults.
5. Government support may shorten the route to success, but a successful campaign can be developed without it.

For the last 2 years, health leaders of twelve Latin American countries, with the support of the International Union Against Cancer, have joined efforts against the colossal enemy the tobacco epidemic represents. Exchange of experience, mutual stimulation, and arousal of interest in neighboring countries are among the goals. The Latin American Coordinating Committee on Smoking Control is the first continental effort toward the tobacco ban. Its example may be useful to other regions of the world.

SUDAN

In 1979, members of the Sudanese Association of Physicians became concerned about the increasing number of diseases attributable to cigarette smoking in men and women, and about the increasing numbers of female adolescent smokers. Members of Parliament and other leading figures were lobbied and, despite the opposition of the tobacco companies, in 1983 a Regulation of Cigarette Smoking Act was passed by the Peoples Assembly. This banned cigarette advertising, controlled smoking in public places, and placed health warnings on cigarette packets. To counter the significant cigarette smuggling problem, the government passed a decree in 1984 to label all cigarette packets "Specially made for Sudan" and all cigarettes "Sudan." The same decree limited the tar content of each cigarette to 15 mg. This prevented the importing of the Marlboro and Benson & Hedges brands, which had higher tar contents.

The tobacco industry fought back. The large posters with the Marlboro cowboy advertising cigarettes were changed to promoting Marlboro lighters. Phillip Morris distributed tee shirts and carrier bags with the Marlboro logo and many shops were painted in the Marlboro colors. Fortunately the government stood firm and these too were abolished. Gallahers responded to the tar content limitation by introducing Sovereign cigarettes with only 15 mg of tar.

In November 1984 the Ministry of Health, supported by the World Health Organization and the International Union Against Cancer organized a Middle East and African Conference on Smoking and Health in Khartoum. There was wide publicity in the newspapers and on radio and television and a great deal of public interest developed, not only on the health consequences of smoking in both men and women but also on the environmental, ecological, cultural, and economic aspects. The conference was a major event for the Sudan in its fight for a smoke-free society, and reinforced the effects of the legislative measures.

Soon after the conference Sudan suffered the full impact of a disastrous famine together with the problem of Civil War in the south of the country. Despite these setbacks, in January 1985 it was decided to initiate the Sudan Anti-Smoking Society (SASS), which was supported not only by doctors but by politicians, artists, teachers, poets, economists, businessmen, and the mass media. There are now rumors that British American Tobacco (BAT) is trying to reintroduce Benson & Hedges cigarettes, and SASS will campaign to prevent this both on health grounds and also to stop the use of precious foreign exchange at a time when the country is suffering such severe food shortages. The Sudanese also plan to prevent the escalation of cigarette smoking which is affecting so many African countries and intend that Sudan should give a powerful example to other Third World countries. In its campaign to combat smoking the Sudan Anti-Smoking Society accepts the challenge to face a powerful and organised industry.

KUWAIT

The health hazards of smoking were recognized in Kuwait as early as 1964, when a smoking control seminar for school health personnel and teachers was organized by the Ministry of Public Health and Ministry of Education. After that seminar, a wide-ranging campaign against smoking was begun, covering schools and youth clubs, as well as the community at large; the media, through the Kuwait radio and television, has also been involved. For example, in 1975 a voluntary agreement was established between the Ministry of Health and owners of public cinemas and theaters to ban tobacco advertisements in these places.

Kuwait also was instrumental in creating an active program against smoking in the Arabian Gulf States. The Smoking Control Committee of the General Health League of Gulf States, which has representatives from the seven Arab states of the Arabian Gulf, has launched a wide-ranging smoking control program including: (1) increasing taxation on imported cigarettes and other tobacco products, (2) limiting tar and nicotine contents to 15 mg of tar and 1 mg of nicotine in imported tobacco products, (3) banning tobacco advertisements in public places and on television, radio, and in the press, (4) printing a health warning on the packages of all cigarettes and other tobacco products, and (5) initiating health education programs about smoking hazards to reach the public through the mass media and the schoolchildren through information in the school curriculum and through an antismoking campaign to be implemented by each school, with activities targeted to children, teachers, and parents. This program has been implemented by the cooperative efforts of the Ministry of Public Health, Ministry of Education, and the Kuwaiti Society for Smoking and Cancer Prevention.

Seminars and workshops for teachers, school nurses, and school social workers include (1) the first Smoking Control Seminar for 800 teachers and other school personnel (in February 1980), (2) the First International Union Against Cancer Regional Smoking Control Workshop for school teachers and children, (3) the First UICC Workshop on Cancer Education in Schools (in December 1983), and (4) inclusion of smoking control courses in the training program of school teachers, nurses, and social workers.

In 1983, the National Smoking Control Week for the public and the private schools included activities such as poster contests for schoolchildren; musical and art performances by children, emphasizing the hazards of smoking; and seminars for schoolchildren and parents. During 1979 (the international Year of the Child), we conducted a survey of schoolchildren from 10 to 14 years of age and found that about 13% of the boys have tried to smoke at least once; less than 6% are regular smokers, most of them above 12 years of age. Another survey of schoolchildren and teachers covered the smoking habits of parents, brothers, and friends of the children. The results showed that about 40% of fathers, 1.7% of mothers, and 38% of brothers are smokers. Incentives were provided for children to persuade parents and other family members who smoke to quit.

AFRICA

Currently, only 10% of African women smoke and they typically begin smoking in their twenties[7] and smoke lightly. Nevertheless, more and more African women are beginning to smoke at a younger age[8] and more heavily. There is no reason to believe that the effects of smoking on reproductive health in Africa will be different from those already seen in developed and other developing countries.[9-11] Clearly there is a case for prevention here, even though the diseases that now predominate in Africa are infections and related to malnutrition.

Historical lessons from developed countries tell us that governments must assume responsibility for smoking control. As reported by Sir George Young, a minister of state of the Conser- vative government of Great Britain in 1979:

> Many of today's medical problems will not be found in the research laboratories of our hospitals but in our parliaments...for the prospective patient the answer may not be cure by incision at the operating table but prevention by decision at the Cabinet table.[12]

The World Health Organization formulated a set of recommendations regarding cigarette production, marketing, and consumption to limit tobacco use. Wickstrom[13] compared these with the policies of seven African countries and found that 86% of the countries adhere to three or fewer of 16 WHO resolutions, 14.0% adhere to between four and eight, and none have implemented more than eight. It is not surprising that in Africa there are generally no warnings on cigarette packs nor are nicotine and tar contents displayed.

Succesful intervention against the increasing use of tobacco in Africa will depend on several factors. First, physicians must educate themselves before they can educate the public, and they must practice what they preach. African physicians need to provide the incontestable facts from the developed and developing worlds to enable health policy makers to make their decisions. They should organize against smoking, in spite of governmental opposition. The short-lived Ghana National Action on Smoking and Health (GNASH) was such an organization. Sudan is initiating such an organization. Second, in smoking control strategies, particularly targeted for adolescents and schoolchildren, the role of pedagogues cannot be overemphasized, as described by Nordgren of Sweden.[14] In Ghana the Ghana Education Service is working on a curriculum incorporating smoking control strategies. The United Nations Educational, Scientific, & Cultural Organization is interested in this project and is providing assistance. Third, education and communication are the keys to success. The perception of the causes of disease is a barrier to be overcome. When the people are made aware of the hazards of smoking by the evidence provided by their physicians, policy makers and executives will begin to listen. Saroso has mentioned the difficulty of making societies besieged by health problems of an environmental nature understand the dangers of chronic disorders from lifestyle.[15] Once that society is learned, it will be able to communicate its concerns to the governments, and all governments, those in khaki or gabardine, those in revolutionary togas and those in indigenous attire, will succumb to pressure from the people and the physicians.

Aggrey of Africa and Ghana, an educator of great eminence, said that educating a man means educating an individual, but educating a woman means educating a nation. African women must be educated about the dangers of cigarette smoking, specifically about the reproductive health hazards. The danger of her loved one getting cancer of the lung or having a heart attack is remote. That she might not conceive a healthy baby, however, will be an immediate concern if she accepts smoking as a possible cause. Thus a vigorous campaign among African women would later be seen as the catalytic force needed for the overall control of smoking in black Africa.

We have just celebrated the success story of the first decade of women; and we have entered the second decade. At the risk of sounding melodramatic, it behooves us all to see that African womanhood does not pass through a smoke-filled tunnel in the next decade or two only to emerge with their lungs lined by anaplastic cells; their coronaries silted with atherosclerotic material, and their wombs in a poor functional state due to the noxious effect of tar, nicotine, benzo(a)pyrene, and hundreds of other substances. Let us resolve that in 10 years we can proclaim another successful decade of African womanhood and not of decayed womanhood.

Acknowledgments

Dr Arabi would like to acknowledge Dr Keith Ball for his contribution in revising the text and his valuable remarks on so many details. He also thanks Miss Huda Gumma, Miss Muna Gadein, and Miss Howayda Motassam for collecting the data and Ibrahim Al Hassan for his analysis.

REFERENCES

1. Luca L, Rigatto M: Epidemiologia do tabagismo: fumo e carboxihemoglobina. *J Pneumologia* 1982;8:146-150.
2. Gross R, Mauad FF, Ruffino Netto, et al: Tabagismo e gravidez: I Prevalencia do habito de fumar entre gestantes. II Repercussoes sobre o produto conceptual. *Rev Assoc Med Bras* 1983;29:4-9.
3. Couto CLM, Castro ES, Rossoni EL, et al: Adolescencia e tabagismo. *Rev Assoc Med R G Sul* 1981;25:26-37.
4. Steglich A, Kauer CL, Martins LHS, et al: *Associacao Anovulatorio—Tabagismo* [monograph]. Porto Alegre, Brazil, Universidade Federal do Rio Grande do Sul, 1983, pp 1-63.
5. Rigatto M: The smoking blossom in developing countries, in *Progress in Smoking Cessation.* New York, American Cancer Society, 1978, pp 66-68.

6. Rigatto M: Expeience in a country without smoking control legislation. Presented at the Fifth World Conference on Smoking and Health, Winnipeg, Man, July 10-15, 1983.
7. Pobee JOM, Larbi EB, Kpodonu J: The profile of the African smoker: The Ghana Smoking Studies. *East Afr Med J* 1984;61: 227-236.
8. Elegbeleye OO, Femi-Pearce D: Incidence and variables contributing to onset of cigarette smoking among secondary school children and medical students in Lagos, Nigeria. *Br J Prev Soc Med* 1976;30:66-70.
9. Jayant K: Tobacco habits in relation to coronary heart disease: a retrospective study in Bombay, India. Presented at WHO Workshop in Colombo [Sri Lanka] on Smoking in Developing Countries. WHO Document Reference WHO/SMO/83, 1981, vol 2, pp 10-16.
10. Jayant K: Information of interest for smoking control programmes in India. Presented at WHO Workshop in Colombo [Sri Lanka] on Smoking in Developing Countries. WHO Document Reference WHO/SMO/83, 1981, vol 2, pp 17-21.
11. Srivastava BN: Profile of smoking in India. Presented at WHO Workshop in Colombo [Sri Lanka] on Smoking in Developing Countries. WHO Document Reference WHO/SMO/83, 1981, vol 2, pp 22-38.
12. Young GS: The politics of smoking, in Ramstrom LM (ed): *The Smoking Epidemic: A Matter of Worldwide Concern.* Proceedings of the Fourth World Congress on Smoking and Health, Stockholm, 1979. Stockholm, Almquist & Wiksell International, 1980.
13. Wickstrom B: Cigarette marketing in the third world—a study of four countries, in Ramstrom LM (ed): *The Smoking Epidemic: A Matter of Worldwide Concern.* Proceedings of the Fourth World Congress on Smoking and Health, Stockholm, 1979. Stockholm, Almquist & Wiksell International, 1980.
14. Nordgren P: Schools and youth organizations, in Ramstrom LM (ed): *The Smoking Epidemic: A Matter of Worldwide Concern.* Proceedings of the Fourth World Congress on Smoking and Health, Stockholm, 1979. Stockholm, Almquist & Wiksell International, 1980.
15. Saroso JS: Possibilities for prevention of smoking associated diseases in developing countries, in Ramstrom LM (ed): *The Smoking Epidemic: A Matter of Worldwide Concern.* Proceedings of the Fourth World Congress on Smoking and Health, Stockholm, 1979. Stockholm, Almquist & Wiksell International, 1980.

35 *The Penalties of Smoking: Low Birth Weight and Increased Neonatal Care Costs*

Gerry Oster, Thomas E. Delea, Graham A. Colditz

Low birth weight is the single most important predictor of neonatal morbidity and death, and infants with low birth weight require significantly greater neonatal intensive care.[1] This suggests that the utilization of neonatal intensive care services may be higher as a result of maternal smoking during pregnancy and that the cost of neonatal care may be greater for infants born to smokers. This paper examines the relationship of maternal smoking during pregnancy to the incidence of low weight births,[2-5] the utilization of neonatal intensive care services, and the economic costs of neonatal care in the United States in 1983.

Although the economic burden of morbidity attributable to cigarette smoking has been considered in earlier studies,[6,7] in none have the costs that arise due to smoking during pregnancy been examined. Although cigarette smoking is linked to a number of adverse outcomes of pregnancy,[8] this analysis is restricted to the effect of smoking on birth weight. In these estimates of the economic burden of an increased number of infants with low birth weight due to smoking, only costs that result from an increase in the number of admissions to neonatal intensive care units (NICUs) have been considered.

METHODS

Estimates of the relative risk of low-weight infants by maternal smoking status[3,9] were combined with data on the prevalence of maternal smoking during pregnancy in the United States[10] to determine the risk attributable to smoking in each of three low birth weight groups (less than 1500 g, 1500-2000 g, and 2000-2500 g). These estimates were multiplied by the total number of liveborn infants in the United States in 1983 in each low birth weight group[11] to estimate the number of infants with low birth weight attributable to maternal smoking during pregnancy.

Probabilities of admission to an NICU for infants in each low birth weight group[12] were used to calculate the number of NICU admissions resulting from maternal smoking. The marginal (or additional) cost per NICU admissions was determined by subtracting the mean charge for routine nursery care[13] from estimates of the median cost of neonatal intensive care in each low birth weight group.[14] All costs are expressed in 1983 dollars according to the medical care component of the Consumer Price Index.[15,16]

These estimates of the additional cost per NICU admission were multiplied by the number of NICU admissions attributable to maternal smoking to yield estimates of the additional cost of neonatal care in each low birth weight group. Summation of these costs across low birth weight groups yields an estimate of the total additional cost of neonatal care attributable to maternal smoking during pregnancy.

The number of liveborn infants in the United States in each birth weight group[11] was multiplied by the probability of NICU admission[12] from infants in that group, then summed across groups to determine the total number of NICU admissions. The total cost of neonatal intensive care in 1983 was calculated by multiplying this estimate by the mean charge (in 1983 dollars) per NICU admission.[14]

RESULTS

In 1983, maternal smoking during pregnancy was responsible for 35,816 births of low weight infants in the United States, or 14.5% of the total number of infants with low birth weight in that year (Table 35-1). Of the estimated 228,297 admissions to NICUs in 1983, 14,978, or 6.6%, were a result of smoking during pregnancy (Table 35-2).

The total neonatal intensive care cost for these infants was $180 million, approximately 5.7% of total national expenditures on neonatal intensive care in 1983. Of this amount, $175 million represents additional costs for care

Table 35-1
The Cost of Neonatal Care Attributable to Maternal Smoking, United States, 1983

Birth Weight Group	Total No. of Low Weight Births[11] (1)	Attributable Risk[3,9,10] (2)	No. of Low Weight Births Attributable to Smoking (3)	Probability of NICU Admission[12] (4)
<1500 g	43,161	.113	4,877	1.00
1501-2000 g	47,309	.119	5,630	.85
2001-2500 g	157,198	.161	25,309	.21
Totals	247,668		35,816	

NICU Admissions Attributable to Smoking (5)	Average Cost per NICU Admission[14-16] (6)	Average Nursery Charge[15,16] (7)	Additional Cost per NICU Admission (8)	Total Additional Cost of Care (9)
4,877	$20,580	$326	$20,254	$99 million
4,786	9,734	326	9,408	45 million
5,315	6,186	326	5,860	31 million
14,978				$175 million

(3) = (1) x (2); (5) = (3) x (4); (8) = (6) - (7); (9) = (5) x (8)

Table 35-2
Maternal Smoking, Low Birth Weight, and Neonatal Intensive Care, United States, 1983

	Low Weight Births (<2500 g)	NICU Admissions	Total NICU Costs
(1) Attributable to Maternal Smoking	35,816	14,978	$180 million
(2) All Births	247,668	228,297	3,157 million
(3) (1) as percent of (2)	14.5%	6.6%	5.7%

that would not have been incurred in the absence of smoking during pregnancy. The cost of neonatal care in the United States in 1983 was therefore $189 higher for infants born to women who smoked during pregnancy than for those born to nonsmoking women.

DISCUSSION

Cigarette smoking during pregnancy imposes a sizeable economic burden on the medical care system, as well as a significant threat to neonatal health. Both nationally and on an individual basis, smoking during pregnancy significantly increases the costs of neonatal care. These findings are even more important when viewed in light of the results of a recent randomized controlled trial, which found that a reduction in smoking during pregnancy significantly increased birth weight over what would be expected if the smoking had been unchanged.[17] Although this analysis does not address the effects of smoking cessation during pregnancy, our findings suggest that the economic benefits of such interventions may be considerable.

Most important among the methodologic limitations of this study is the fact that our analysis is retrospective and based on data from a variety of sources. The validity of our findings therefore depends on the internal and external validity of the studies on which the analysis is based. Although we have attempted to control for sources of bias in our estimates through the selective use of available secondary data, some bias may remain and the estimates may consequently lack precision.

In particular, because the risk of low birth weight has been linked to a number of factors in addition to cigarette smoking—eg, socioeconomic status, height, maternal age, and prepregnancy weight—estimates of relative risk are used that are based on a multivariate analysis of the relationship between smoking and low birth weight in the population of the Collaborative Perinatal Project of the National Institute of Neurological and Communicative Diseases and Stroke.[9] Accordingly, the estimates of relative and attributable risk depend on the representativeness of this study population, as well as the accuracy with which the true relationship between smoking during pregnancy and low birth weight was modeled in this earlier study.

Estimates of the likelihood of admission to an NICU by weight at birth were taken from a 13-county study of prenatal care among MediCal recipients in California.[12] Patterns of care may differ for those who are not participants in this program or those who reside outside the study area, and our estimates of the number of NICU admissions attributable to maternal smoking may accordingly be biased. Perhaps more important, the likelihood of NICU admission is assumed to depend only on birth weight and to be independent of maternal smoking status. If small-for-gestational age infants born to women who smoke experience less morbidity at any given birth weight than do infants born to nonsmoking women, the number of NICU admissions attributable to maternal smoking would be overestimated.

Estimates of costs per NICU admission come from a study of admissions to the intensive care nursery at the University of California, San Francisco,[14] and are not representative of costs in all settings. These estimates were also based on data for hospital charges and hence may overstate the actual resource costs of neonatal care. In addition, these data are more than a decade old, and, although they were inflated for changes in the Consumer Price Index for medical care, they could not be adjusted specifically for changes in the cost of care due to changes in neonatal intensive care technology.

Despite these limitations, this estimate of the cost of neonatal care attributable to maternal smoking during pregnancy is conservative, since only the effect of maternal smoking on low birth weight is considered and other complications of pregnancy linked to cigarette smoking are excluded. Nor are the long-term effects of smoking during pregnancy on childhood health considered.

Despite the conservative nature of our estimates, these results highlight the effect of smoking during pregnancy on neonatal health. By drawing attention to the relationship between maternal smoking and the costs of neonatal care, we may heighten the interest of health care providers in interventions to reduce this burden.

Acknowledgments

The author appreciates the assistance of Enriqueta Bond, PhD; James G. Hill; Joel C. Kleinman, PhD; Carol C. Korenbrot, PhD; Peggy McManus, MHS; Ciaran S. Phipps, BA; John Pinney, BA; Paul J. Placek, PhD; Douglas Richardson, MD; Mary Sexton, PhD, MPH; and Peter Thexton.

REFERENCES

1. Budetti P, McManus P, Barrand N, et al: The cost and effectiveness of neonatal intensive care. Office of Technology Assessment, US Congress, 1981.

2. US Dept of Health and Human Services: *Smoking and Health. A report of the Surgeon General.* US Dept of Public Health, Education and Welfare publication No. (PHS) 79-50066, Government Printing Office, 1979.
3. McMahon B, Alpert M, Salbert EJ: Infant weight and parental smoking habits. *Am J Epidemiol* 1966;82:247-261.
4. Meyer MB, Comstock GW: Maternal cigarette smoking and perinatal mortality. *Am J Epidemiol* 1972;96:1-10.
5. Yerushalmy J: The relationship of parents' cigarette smoking to outcome of pregnancy--implications as to the problem of inferring causation from observed associations. *Am J Epidemiol* 1971;93:443-455.
6. Oster G, Colditz GA, Kelly NL: The economic costs of smoking and the benefits of quitting for individual smokers. *Prev Med* 984;13:377-389.
7. Luce BR, Schweitzer SO: Smoking and alcohol abuse: a comparison of the economic consequences. *N Engl J Med* 1978;298:569-571.
8. Meyer MB, Jonas BS, Tonascia JA: Perinatal events associated with maternal smoking during pregnancy. *Am J Epidemiol* 1976;103:464-476.
9. Nelson KB, Ellenberg JH: Predictors of low and very low birth weight and the relation of these to cerebral palsy. *JAMA* 1985;254:1473-1479.
10. National Center for Health Statistics: *Health, United States, 1983.* US Dept of Health and Human Services publication No. (PHS) 84-1232, 1983.
11. National Center for Health Statistics: *Advance Report of Final Natality Statistics, 1983. Monthly Vital Statistics Report,* vol 34, No. 6 suppl, Sept 20, 1985. US Dept of Health and Human Services publication No. (PHS) 85-1120, 1985.
12. Korenbrot CC: Risk reduction in pregnancies of low-income women. Comprehensive prenatal care through the OB access project. *Mobius* 1984;4:34-43.
13. *The Cost of Having a Baby.* Washington, Health Insurance Association of America,1983.
14. Phibbs CS, Williams RL, Phibbs RH: Newborn risk factors and the cost of neonatal intensive care. *Pediatrics* 1981;68:313-321.
15. *Consumer Price Index, Detailed Report, October 1977.* US Dept of Labor, Bureau of Labor Statistics, 1977.
16. *Consumer Price Index, Detailed Report. December 1983.* US Department of Labor, Bureau of Labor Statistics, 1984.
17. Sexton M, Hebel JR: A clinical trial of change in maternal smoking and its effect on birth weight. *JAMA* 1984;25:911-915.

36 *How to Help the Pregnant Woman Stop Smoking*

Susan Wilner, R.H. Secker-Walker, B.S. Flynn, L.J. Solomon, L. Collins-Burris, S. LePage, B.V. McPherson, P. Mead, Elaine Bratic Arkin, Karen Monaco, Dee Burton

The challenge facing all who provide health services to women of reproductive age is how to help them stop smoking. Approximately a third of all pregnant women in the United States smoke, which means that each year at least 1 million babies are unnecessarily exposed to the health hazards of smoking. Several population-based studies have demonstrated that about 25% of pregnant smokers stop for a reason related to their pregnancy.[1-3] Ample evidence also suggests that another 20% to 25% could be assisted with appropriate intervention.[4] However, nearly 80% of women who stop smoking during pregnancy will relapse anywhere from one hour to 1 year postpartum. Thus, an additional challenge is how to help these women sustain their initial success. This paper reviews a series of options aimed at encouraging pregnant women to stop smoking, including discussion of preliminary results of several intervention studies, the role of various organizations with this common goal, and a notable advertising approach.

INTERVENTION EFFORTS

A 1984 review[4] indicates that most smoking cessation studies incorporate one or more of the most common forms of intervention techniques used in health promotion programs: counseling, groups, self-help materials, and information supplied through the media.[5-12] Several approaches described in the literature review can aid practitioners in establishing effective strategies. Perhaps most important is counseling by a woman's physician or other primary-care clinician, which appears to be among the most effective intervention strategies for the pregnant smoker.[13] Group counseling programs, self-help materials, and mass media advertisements are useful adjuncts for pregnant smokers, but should not be used as the primary modality. Social support (from spouses, partners, or other family members) appears to be a critical factor in changing smoking behavior. Since nearly 80% of those who quit during pregnancy relapse within a year, repeated messages appear to be necessary to sustain behavior changes. Additional evaluation of this strategy is needed. Methods to reach high-risk groups (such as pregnant teen-agers) and to disseminate existing programs are also needed.

Partly in response to this review, the National Academy of Science's Committee to Study the Prevention of Low Birth Weight issued the following summary report:

> The committee urges that helping women to stop or reduce smoking in pregnancy become a major concern of obstetric care providers. Research to define how best to address the smoking problem should receive high priority; simultaneously, antismoking advice should be offered routinely by physicians and other maternity care providers and supplemented, where possible, by educational materials, mediabased messages, and related strategies.14

HOW TO IMPLEMENT A PROGRAM

In late 1984, the design for a smoking intervention strategy for pregnant women attending neighborhood health centers in Massachusetts was initiated.[7] The challenge was to develop a system that could be implemented in most of the 19 centers, which serve a variety of population groups, including low-income, teen-aged, and single parents.

An assessment of the providers' needs revealed that they felt they needed more information and skills on how to counsel their patients effectively, a reminder system to initiate the counseling process at each prenatal visit, and written materials for patients as support and reinforcement of the providers' message. Based on this information, a three-part system for the intervention strategy was designed which included a provider training program, a medical-record reminder system, and patient education materials. Providers were encouraged to follow four simple steps, and an acronym was formed to help them remember this approach: *STOP* for *S*ympathize; *T*ake a smoking history; *O*ffer information; and *P*ropose a quitting date.

The booklet *Quitting for You 2* was written to be distributed by providers to patients at the first prenatal visit and to reinforce the provider's message to stop smoking. The book was written to be upbeat in tone and to suggest positive substitute behaviors for smoking, rather than the more traditional techniques of arousing fear and guilt. This (or any other book) is recommended only as an adjunct to and never a substitute for effective and consistent counseling by a health care provider at each prenatal visit.

The project's pilot phase has now been completed. The system designed was easily implemented in the neighborhood health centers and utilized by their staff. A report on this project documents the findings more completely.[7] The program described is just one of many efforts under way nationally, which are helping the more than 1 million women each year who smoke during pregnancy. These efforts will help achieve the objectives for the nation of improving the health of mothers and newborn infants.

CESSATION COUNSELING DURING OBSTETRIC CARE

A randomized controlled trial of smoking cessation counseling during obstetric care has been in progress at the University of Vermont since May 1984. Women assigned to the intervention program are counseled a minimum of five times during their pre- and postnatal clinic visits. Women in the "usual care" group are given the American Lung Association (ALA) pamphlet on smoking and pregnancy. The following is a summary of the experience of the first 139 women who had completed a visit at 36 weeks of pregnancy by September 1985.

There was a significant decrease in cigarette consumption in the intervention group, but not in the control group. The quit rates were similar: 15.2% in the intervention group and 13.7% in the controls. Cigarettes smoked per day at first visit, expressed intentions of stopping, and number of previous attempts to stop were all significantly related to both changing smoking behavior and quitting by the 36th week of pregnancy. Only 15.7% of the variance in quitting was explained by these three variables and the variables of age and overall motivation to stop smoking.

Cigarettes smoked per day and expressed intention to quit were the best predictors of quitting smoking[15-17]; expressed intention to quit can be increased by physicians' advice to stop smoking.[18] Predictors of a favorable response to intervention will be a focus of further analyses.

HEALTHY MOTHERS, HEALTHY BABIES: A NATIONAL COALITION

The National Healthy Mothers, Healthy Babies Coalition was founded in 1981 to promote preventive health habits for all pregnant women and their families by developing education materials and networks to distribute them. The coalition provides the opportunity to begin to make changes within the many women's (and other) organizations that have no smoking policies or programs.

An executive secretariat in Washington, DC, manages the coalition, whose members include about 70 national professional, governmental, and voluntary organizations (including the American College of Obstetricians and Gynecologists, Salvation Army, and the National Association of Counties). Six subcommittees address the following priorities: substance abuse during pregnancy; breast-feeding; genetic screening; oral health; low income women; and adolescent pregnancy. Basic educational materials incorporate messages about smoking and pregnancy, alcohol and drug use, nutrition, breast-feeding, and prenatal care.

Unfortunately, more is needed than just opening these new channels for communication. In 1985 the Low Income Subcommittee found that almost none of 1500 health care providers surveyed reported counseling pregnant women about the hazards of smoking, emphasizing the need for more work in traditional health care areas. In the past year a resource packet produced in co-operation with the American Lung Association and many other organizations on alcohol, cigarette, and drug use during pregnancy was sent to about 20,000 health care providers who work with pregnant women.

The National Coalition is participating in the Office on Smoking and Health's mass media campaign on smoking and pregnancy. More than 4 million television, radio, poster, and pamphlet messages have been distributed in less than 6 months. In addition, ten state coalitions (which the national coalition is dedicated to developing) are planning statewide mass media campaigns about smoking, nutrition, and prenatal care. The opportunity exists to greatly expand smoking programs and therefore to help mothers have healthier babies through these 70 national organizations and more than 40 state coalitions.

THE AMERICAN LUNG ASSOCIATION: THE ROLE OF A VOLUNTARY AGENCY

Although the ALA discouraged smoking during pregnancy for many years with its own smoking and pregnancy program, in 1983 it joined the Healthy Mothers, Healthy Babies Coalition. A major reason for this collaboration was to determine how to better educate health care providers about smoking counseling for pregnant women, but several other programs and projects have resulted.

The ALA worked with the March of Dimes and the National Cancer Institute to provide and distribute smoking cessation booklets for Hispanics. Working with Harvard Community Health Plan, ALA developed a self-help smoking cessation manual, "Freedom from Smoking® for You and Your Baby." Collaboration appears to carry more clout than a single-agency effort in reducing the smoking and pregnancy problem.

The "Smoking Fetus": A Case Study in Pro-Health Advertising

There is a need for mass media promotion of smoking cessation among pregnant women. Twenty-one percent of pregnant women are unaware of smoking's harmful effects on the fetus.[19] In a study of black and Mexican-American pregnant women performed as part of the "Healthy Mother" project 54% of the health care providers reported that women need but do not seek information on smoking's effects on pregnancy.[20] Mass media approaches are particularly useful for reaching such an audience, where a need exists without apparent desire for information. The "Smoking Fetus" ad, as it came to be known, was designed to reach this audience.

Effective mass media programs tend to have certain common characteristics. They usually know their audience and rely most heavily on the medium most used by their target population. For pregnant women the appropriate medium is television, according to the 1982 survey of exposure to print and electronic media (US Dept of Health and Human Services, unpublished data). Television is also a medium of high exposure for people in low socioeconomic environments, where many smokers tend to be. Effective programs deliver compelling messages that prompt or reinforce interpersonal communication. It is largely the combined effect of media efforts, together with conversations with friends, family members, and health care professionals, that lead to behavior change. Finally, advertisements that have substantial impact are typically easily recognizable in form and simple in content.

The "Smoking Fetus" (Figure 36-1) delivers needed information to the specifically targeted group of pregnant women by using the most appropriate medium, television. It appeals in both sight and sound and is simple and compelling. It is an antiproduct ad (the product is shown to contradict something of value) like most other antismoking ads. When the "Smoking Fetus" was offered through the American Cancer Society to the major television networks, ABC accepted it but NBC and CBS refused to air it on the grounds that it was too graphic and might offend some viewers. Ironically, these refusals sparked a controversy that resulted in the ad's being shown on all three networks on talk shows.

The issue about whether fear-arousal is an appropriate route to promote smoking cessation among pregnant women is controversial. Although it has long been considered in the health education field that using scare tactics should be avoided, in his review of 44 studies, Sutton[21] found that fear-arousal communications are effective. Fear-arousal in the "Smoking Fetus," then, is an additional characteristic that should prove effective in promoting smoking cessation.

The "Smoking Fetus" (its official title is "Mothers, Please Don't Smoke") was created by Joseph Vogt and is the winner of, among other awards, a Sweepstakes Award of the American Advertising Federation Best in the West awards; 1st Place, Public Service category of the Peninsula Press Club; a Gold Award for Public Service from the San Francisco Advertising Club Cable Car awards; a World's Best Television Public Service Announcement, 1984, from the Hollywood Radio & Television Society, International Broadcasting awards; a Certificate of Achievement for Excellence in Television Advertising from Advertising Age magazine, a Certificate of Creative Excellence and Recognition for Public Service from the 1985 Clio Awards; a Gold Award from the San Francisco Art Directors Club, and a Special Jury Award from the Houston International Film Festival.

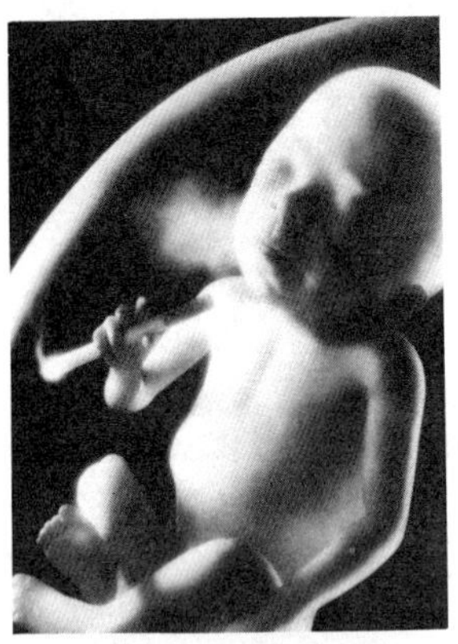

PREGNANT MOTHERS: PLEASE DON'T SMOKE!

If you are pregnant or planning a family, here are three good reasons to quit smoking now:

1. Smoking retards the growth of your baby in your womb.

2. Smoking increases the incidence of infant mortality.

3. Your family needs a healthy mother.

Please don't smoke for your baby's sake.

And yours.

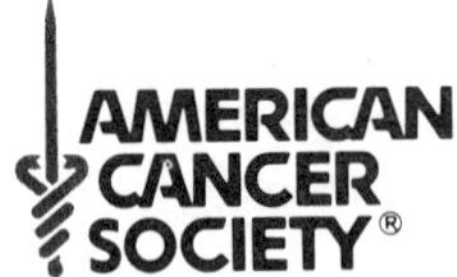

Figure 36-1

SUMMARY

In describing these varied approaches, it is hoped that professionals around the country will be encouraged to implement new cessation program initiatives for pregnant smokers in their communities. The state of the art in this field is such that there are a number of excellent programs ready for dissemination and implementation. The Centers for Disease Control will be issuing a monograph later this year entitled *Planning and Evaluation of Smoking Cessation Programs for Pregnant Women,* which will summarize these programs.

REFERENCES

1. Kuzma SW, Kissinger DG: Patterns of alcohol and cigarette use in pregnancy. *Neurol Toxicol Teratol* 1981;3:211-221.
2. Prager K, Malin H, Spiegler D, et al: Smoking and drinking behavior before and during pregnancy. *Public Health Rep* 1984;99:117-127.
3. Wilner S, Schoenbaum S, Palmer RH, et al: Smoking and quitting during pregnancy: Who does and who doesn't, in *Maternity Care in Two Health Care Systems.* Harvard University School of Public Health, Cambridge, Mass, doctoral dissertation, 1981.
4. Wilner S: *A Summary of Efforts to Reduce Smoking Among Pregnant Women.* Commissioned report for the Committee to Study the Prevention of Low Birthweight, Institute of Medicine, Washington, National Academy of Sciences, 1984.
5. Donovan J: Randomized controlled trial of anti-smoking advice in pregnancy. *Br J Prev Soc Med* 1977;31:6-12.
6. Sexton M, Hebel JR: A clinical trial of change in maternal smoking and its effect on birthweight. *JAMA* 1984;251:911-915.
7. Wilner S, Blatt JR, Naah S: *Quitting for You 2.* The Massachusetts Department of Public Health Smoking Intervention Program. Boston, Division of Maternal and Child Health, 1985.
8. Windsor RA, Cutter G, Morris J, et al: The effectiveness of smoking cessation methods for smokers in public health maternity clinics: a randomized trial. *Am J Public Health* 1985;75:1389-1392.
9. Ershoff DH, Aaronson NK, Danaher BG, et al: Behavioral, health and cost outcomes of an HMO-based prenatal health education program. *Public Health Rep* 1983;98:536-542.
10. Loeb BK, Bailey JW, Waage G, et al: A randomized trial of smoking intervention during pregnancy. Presented at Fifth World Conference on Smoking and Health, Winnepeg, Man, July 10-15, 1983.
11. Bigelow G., Robinson C, Mead A: Changes in smoking during pregnancy. Presented at the meeting of the Society for Behavioral Medicine, Philadelphia, May 1984.
12. Li VC, Coates T, Spielberg L, et al: Smoking cessation with young women in public family planning clinics: the impact of physician messages and waiting room media. *Prev Med* 1984;13:472-489.
13. American Lung Association: *Smoking and Pregnancy: Handbook for Health Care Providers,* New York, 1982, p 7.

14. Institute of Medicine. *Committee to Study the Prevention of Low Birthweight. Preventing Low Birthweight.* Institute of Medicine, National Academy Press, 1985, pp 184-187.
15. Li VC, Kim J, Ewar C, et al: Effects of physician counseling on smoking behavior of asbestos-exposed workers. *Prev Med* 1984;13:462-476.
16. Li VC, Contes T, Spielberg L, et al: Smoking cessation with young women in public family planning clinics: The impact of physician messages and waiting room media. *Prev Med* 1984;13:459-477.
17. Pederson LL: Compliance with physician advice to quit smoking: A review of the literature. *Prev Med* 1982;11:71-84.
18. Russell MAH, Wilson C, Taylor C, et al: Effect of general practitioner's advice against smoking. *Br Med J* 1979;2:231-235.
19. Black P: Who stops smoking in pregnancy? *Nursing Times* 1984;80:59-61.
20. Juarez & Associates, Inc: *"Healthy Mothers" Market Research: How to Reach Black and Mexican American Women.* Report submitted to US Dept of Health and Human Services, contract No. 282-81-0082, Sept 14, 1982.
21. Sutton SR: Fear-arousal communications: a critical examination of theory and research, in Eiser JR (ed): *Social Psychology and Behavioral Medicine.* New York, John Wiley & Sons, 1982, pp 303-337.

37 *Postpartum Smoking*

Mary Sexton, J. Richard Hebel, Norma Lynn Fox

We have found that smoking cessation intervention during pregnancy can improve the quit rate by at least twofold.[1] Less clear, however, is whether women who quit smoking during pregnancy—with or without assistance—maintain abstinence after delivery of the child. To address this issue, the recidivism rates over a 3-year period were analyzed for a cohort of Maryland women who participated in a randomized clinical trial of smoking cessation intervention during pregnancy.

This trial was designed to test the hypothesis that a reduction in maternal smoking during pregnancy would result in an increase in the birth weight of the infant. Over a 2 1/2-year period, 935 pregnant smokers were identified when they registered for prenatal care and were randomly allocated, usually in the 15th week of pregnancy, to a control group or to a treatment group. The treatment group was given special assistance and encouragement to quit smoking. When they were assigned to the treatment or control group and again at the eighth month of pregnancy, women reported their smoking habits and provided a sample of saliva for measurement of thiocyanate, a biochemical indicator of smoking.[1] The smoking cessation intervention significantly increased the percentage of women who quit smoking. Only 20% of the control group had quit smoking by the eighth month; in contrast, 43% of the treatment group had quit. More importantly, this increase in smoking cessation resulted in a significant increase in birth weight.[1,2] The results of the pregnancy outcome study and sociodemographic characteristics have been described previously.[1,2]

In examining recidivism, we analyzed the woman's smoking status at 3 months and 3 years after delivery (Table 37-1). The 86 baseline quitters (women who quit before prenatal care) were relatively successful in abstaining from smoking throughout pregnancy; 84% (32/38) of the baseline quitters in the treatment group were nonsmokers at the eighth month of pregnancy, but 25% (12/48) of the baseline quitters in the control group had resumed smoking. At 3 months after delivery, more than half of the baseline quitters in the treatment and control groups had resumed smoking. Further deterioration in the quit rates took place over time, but not as much as in the interval between late pregnancy and 3 months after delivery. Assignment to the treatment (intervention) group did not help the baseline quitters sustain their quitting after the child was born. Intervention during pregnancy seemed to assist in a small way in preventing recidivism before the pregnancy ended; it did not help, however, in maintaining abstinence and may have even increased the probability of resuming smoking after delivery.

Women who were smokers when they registered for prenatal care averaged 14 cigarettes per day at the time of registration. By the eighth month of pregnancy, only 7% of the control group (given only the usual influence from obstetricians, other health personnel, and family and friends) had stopped smoking. In contrast, a third of the women in the treatment group were able to quit. Assistance given as a part of the usual obstetric and prenatal care was relatively ineffective in helping women to quit smoking. The intervention by the project staff[3] was modest in intensity. However, even this modest level of assistance did improve smoking cessation and pregnancy outcome. The babies in the treatment group showed a significant reduction in fetal growth retardation.

These results underscore the need for including smoking cessation assistance as a part of the routine prenatal care protocol. Overall, however, a very high percentage resumed smoking; 81% of the treatment group and 88% of the control group smoked at 3 months after delivery. This small but statistically significant difference between the treatment and control groups was lost by the third year after delivery. Furthermore, the women resumed their smoking at about the level they had smoked prior to pregnancy.

We also examined smoking status during subsequent pregnancies. Twenty-four percent of the previous baseline quitters and 74% of the previous baseline smokers reported smoking for more than 6 months during the pregnancy following the index pregnancy. These data show that if nonsmoking in

TABLE 37-1
Smoking Cessation Rates For Women Who Did And Did Not Smoke At Enrollment

Percentage of Nonsmokers During Pregnancy	"Baseline Quitters"*		Smokers at Time of Prenatal Registration	
	Treatment Group (n = 38)	Control Group (n = 48)	Treatment Group (n = 300)	Control Group (n = 313)
Eighth month of pregnancy				
Quit rates	84%	75%	32%	7%†
Mean No. of cigarettes/day	1.1	2.4	8.2	15.6
Abstinence rates after delivery				
	Treatment Group (n = 36)	Control Group (n = 47)	Treatment Group (n = 298)	Control Group (n = 312)
Three months after delivery				
Abstinence rates	46%	49%	19%	12%§
No. of cigarettes/day	NA	NA	NA	NA
	Treatment Group (n = 38)	Control Group (n = 48)	Treatment Group (n = 298)	Control Group (n = 312)
Three years after delivery				
Abstinence rates	37%	42%	11%	9%
No. of cigarettes/day	18.2	16.6	19.0	19.8

Quit Rates *During* Pregnancy for Those Smoking at Time of Prenatal Care (N=61

	Treatment Group (n = 302)	Control Group (n = 314)
During Pregnancy		
At enrollment (av 15-wk gestation)		
Quit rates	0%	0%
Mean No. of cigarettes/day	13.1	15.0
Eighth month of pregnancy		
Quit rates	32%	7%†
Mean No. of cigarettes/day	8.2	15.6

NA = not available.
*Smokers who quit prior to prenatal registration.
† $P \leq .01$
§ $P < .05$.

pregnancy is to be sustained, there must be assistance with maintenance after delivery. Moreover, this assistance should be initiated very early, preferably before the woman and baby leave the hospital. Clearly, the intervention has to prepare women to counter the high risk of resuming smoking after delivery.

These data point to the need for developing and providing effective smoking cessation assistance during pregnancy and the postpartum period. Of the maternal characteristics that put a pregnancy at risk, maternal smoking is one that is highly prevalent, with about a third of the women entering their pregnancies as smokers and only about a fourth of those being able to quit on their own. In other words, about one out of four pregnancies undergoes risk until term because of maternal smoking.

High alcohol intake before the pregnancy, low parity, and being a clinic patient were the best predictors of recidivism, whether the baseline factors were examined singly or in a multiple logistic regression model. In the model, prepregnancy alcohol use, parity, and being a clinic patient each made a significant contribution when the data were adjusted for all other relevant factors.

Since the labor and delivery factors did not influence the recidivism rates at 3 months, it is not surprising that there was no relationship with the 3-year smoking status. Being a patient at a clinic, being black, having a lower level of education, and being younger were related to resuming smoking. No clinical or behavioral factor was associated with the resumption of smoking. When all factors were entered into a stepwise regression model, only one factor—being a clinic patient—retained significance ($P < .10$). The baseline level of smoking during pregnancy did not relate to abstinence after delivery. Similar to findings from other studies, we found that the amount of smoking at baseline in this cohort was significantly related to smoking late in pregnancy, when other factors were controlled. Many other studies have found that the less a person smokes, the more likely she will be to quit smoking. Thus, the lack of a relationship with postpartum recidivism was not anticipated.

One possible explanation for the discrepancy in the relationship between the baseline and pregnancy smoking levels and the baseline and postpartum smoking levels is that the cohort of quitters might be more homogeneous with respect to smoking and other behaviors. These quitters, for example, were smoking fewer than nine cigarettes at baseline, compared with 14 cigarettes for all women who were smoking at the time of registration. The women met several criteria before they were included in the recidivism analysis. They were smoking at the time of prenatal care registration, they stopped later in pregnancy, and their pregnancies resulted in single liveborn infants. Therefore, the truncated distribution with respect to amount of smoking may be the reason that baseline smoking did not relate to recidivism.

In summary, the data from the Maryland cohort strongly suggest that smoking intervention programs limited to prenatal contacts can be effective in increasing the percentage of smokers who quit during a given pregnancy. They do not, however, have any holding power for helping women achieve long-term abstinence or helping them abstain during a subsequent pregnancy.

REFERENCES

1. Sexton M, Hebel JR: A clinical trial of change in maternal smoking and its effect on birth weight. *JAMA* 1984;251:911-915.
2. Hebel JR, Nowicki P, Sexton M: The effect of antismoking intervention during pregnancy: an assessment of interactions with maternal characteristics. *Am J Epidemiol* 1985;122:135-148.
3. Nowicki P, Gintzig L, Hebel JR, et al: Effective smoking intervention during pregnancy. *Birth* 1984;11:217-224.

38 *Funding Smoking Cessation Activities and Research: The NIH Experience*

Thomas J. Glynn

Four institutes in the National Institutes of Health (NIH) have, or are developing, a significant involvement in smoking and tobacco use—the National Cancer Institute (NCI), the National Heart, Lung, and Blood Institute (NHLBI), the National Institute of Child Health and Human Development (NICHHD), and the National Institute of Dental Research (NIDR). The NHLBI supports and conducts research related to the effects of smoking on the respiratory and cardiovascular system. The NICHD supports research on the psychosocial antecedents of cigarette smoking in children and adolescents and on helping pregnant women reduce or eliminate smoking. The NIDR supports research focusing on the role of smokeless tobacco in dental and orofacial diseases and conditions.[1] The Smoking, Tobacco, and Cancer Program (STCP) of the National Cancer Institute will be described in detail because it is the largest and most centralized of the NIH smoking programs and may serve as a prototype for programs in other areas of the United States as well as other countries.

Having begun in late 1982, the STCP is a relatively new program in the NCI. Prior to that time, the NCI had focused on establishing tobacco's role in cancer etiology (pre-1975) and on developing a less hazardous cigarette (from 1975 to around 1981). However, with the development of a centralized tobacco research program in 1982, the STCP now serves as the focal point for the NCI's research, disease prevention, and health promotion activities related to tobacco use and cancer.

The goal of the STCP is straightforward: to decrease the incidence of cancer caused by or related to smoking and the use of tobacco products. Although the essential activities of basic research, information dissemination, and surveillance and evaluation will continue, the primary means by which this goal is being addressed is through a program of controlled intervention trials, based on sound biomedical and behavioral research findings. Each of these trials is intended to develop cost-effective, durable, widely applicable, and readily adoptable interventions that will aid specific target populations to either stop or not start smoking.

The STCP is supporting intervention trials in six major areas: adolescent smoking prevention, developing self-help smoking cessation strategies, utilizing physicians and dentists as interveners, developing mass media approaches to smoking prevention and cessation, and prevention and cessation of smoking among US black and Hispanic populations. During the next 5 years, the activities of the STCP will contribute to the NCI goal of reducing cancer mortality by 50% by the year 2000 and provide the means by which smoking-related cancer incidence will be reduced after the year 2000. These activities include: completing the intervention trials; expanding to include research on prevention and cessation of smoking among women, intervention for smokeless tobacco users, and cessation methods for heavy smokers; development of a collaborative smoking intervention research network; and initiating a smoking research applications program to promote and utilize proven prevention and cessation strategies.

Although active intramural research programs deal with tobacco in all the relevant NIH Institutes, most of the research resources in this area go to extramural investigators. In 1985, for example, the smoking-related research budgets of the relevant institutes were:

National Cancer Institute	$20.4 million
National Heart, Lung, and Blood Institute	8.2 million
National Institute of Child Health and HumanDevelopment	2.6 million
National Institute on Drug Abuse	3.0 million
TOTAL	$34.2 million

Research with these funds is distributed and carried out in a number of ways.

Award mechanisms The NIH research and development award mechanisms are divided into three basic categories: grants, cooperative agreements, and contracts. Most applications for grant support are originated by an individual investigator who develops a research proposal in an area of interest to the federal program. In addition, program announcements and requests for applications (RFAs) are published to stimulate submission of applications in areas of high priority or special concern. Generally, program announcements describe new, continuing, or expanded program interests, or announce the availability of a new mechanism of support. The RFAs invite grant applications in a well-defined area to accomplish a specific program purpose.

Cooperative agreements are similar to grants in that they are a mechanism to assist and support research. They are used whenever substantial federal involvement with the recipient during performance of the research is anticipated. Federal involvement may include assisting recipients in carrying out projects or reviewing and approving certain phases of the projects. Application, review, and administration of cooperative agreements are similar to those for grants. An important difference, however, is that a specific program announcement or RFA describing the nature of the federal involvement must be issued. In the past, only public and private nonprofit organizations were eligible for grant and cooperative agreement funding. Profit-making organizations are now eligible for grant and cooperative agreement funding as well as for contract funding.

The initiative for research and development contracts usually comes from NIH staff. Notices of requests for proposals (RFPs) are published in the *Commerce Business Daily*. Notices of NIH solicitations usually appear in the *NIH Guide for Grants and Contracts*, as well. Contract performance is closely monitored by program staff to ensure accomplishment of project goals for the benefit of or use by the awarding federal program. Most programs in the NIH also participate in the Small Business Innovation Research Program.

Within the broad grant mechanism, the major categories are:

1. Research project grants, which are the basic grant mechanisms used in the NIH. They are awarded to institutions on behalf of individual investigators.
2. New investigator research awards, which support basic and clinical studies conducted by newly trained investigators or investigators addressing a field new to them.
3. Program project grants, which support broadly based, often multidisciplinary, long-term research programs with a particular major objective or theme.
4. Center grants, which support long-term, multidisciplinary programs of research and development. Center grants are more likely to have a clinical orientation than are program project grants, and

proposals are developed in response to the specific needs of an institute.

5. Small grants of no more than $35,000, which are awarded primarily to new investigators. Small grants, which are short-term and may not be renewed, may support pilot studies or the development and testing of new methods.

6. Research scientist development awards, which support scientists who need advanced research training or additional experience to enable them to engage in full time and long-term research.

7. Research career development awards, which support individuals in the formative stages of their careers who have demonstrated outstanding potential for contributing as independent investigators to health-related research.

8. Clinical investigator awards, which provide research support to individuals with clinical training or experience and demonstrated aptitude, who are potential independent investigators. These awards are intended to fill gaps among faculty of health professional institutions.

9. Conference grant awards, which provide a portion of the cost of a conference relevant to a particular institute.

Application and Review Procedures The NIH grant applications are processed through the Division of Research Grants (DRG) at NIH. Application kits may be obtained from the Division of Research Grants, 5333 Westbard Ave, National Institutes of Health, Bethesda, MD 20893. Frequently, institutional grant and contract offices maintain supplies of these kits. Care should be taken to ensure that the most recent application kit is used; they are updated frequently, and proposals submitted on out-of-date forms may be disallowed. Grant applications are also submitted to the Division of Research Grants.

In the Division of Research Grants, an application is assigned to both an initial review group (IRG) for scientific merit review and to a particular bureau, institute, or division for possible funding. Applications are subjected to a two-level review process. The first level of review is performed by IRGs, which are composed primarily of nonfederal scientists with expertise in specific scientific areas. An NIH staff member serves as executive secretary of the review group. In assessing the scientific and technical merit of the applications, the IRGs consider the scientific and technical significance and the originality of the proposed research, the adequacy of the method, the qualifications and experience of the investigator(s), the suitability of the facilities, and the appropriateness of the budget requested.

For each application, the IRG votes to recommend approval, disapproval, or deferral for additional information. The second level of application review is made by the national advisory council of the bureau, institute, or division. The council, which is composed of scientific and lay members, receives all proposals, their priority scores, and the executive secretary's summary reports of the review group's deliberations. The advisory council considers the recommendation of the review group and makes its own evaluation of the proposal's relevance to the institute's overall goals. An award is made only if the application has been recommended for approval by the national advisory council and if the priority score is within the range determined by the institute's budget and program needs.

Solicited contract proposals are usually evaluated by nonfederal scientists against fixed evaluation criteria specified in the RFP. In addition, program staff provide separate evaluations of the cost proposals. Funding decisions are based on recommendations of the scientific reviewers and staff budget evaluations. Advisory councils or boards are not required to approve individual contract projects, although these councils and boards are involved in an institute's overall program and research planning, which includes allocating resources for both grants and contracts.[2]

SMOKING-RELATED RESEARCH DIRECTIONS

Current basic research initiatives, such as investigations of the carcinogenicity of new tobacco products, the synergistic effects of tobacco and other carcinogens, the use of smokeless tobacco, and the risk involved in involuntary/passive smoking, as well as the intervention research initiatives discussed above, will continue. How will these change? What new tobacco-related research initiatives can be expected in the future?

Although the importance of the tobacco and health issue makes a wide range of research desirable, the inevitable limits on resources make choices necessary. As a result, the following are likely to be the research directions of this field in the near future:

1. Developing more effective systems for monitoring current trends and new uses of tobacco products
2. Developing a wide array of smoking prevention/cessation interventions demonstrated to be effective in defined population studies.
3. Developing valid methods for monitoring the effects of policies and activities (eg, taxes, local ordinances, advertising) thought to affect smoking and tobacco use incidence and prevalence.
4. Developing strategies for effective dissemination, diffusion, and utilization of successful smoking interventions.

REFERENCES

1. National Institutes of Health, Division of Research Grants: *Referral Guidelines for Funding Components of the Public Health Service*, Government Printing Office, 1985.
2. Dusek ER, Holt VE, Burke ME, et al (eds): *The American Psychological Association's Guide to Research Support*, Washington, American Psychological Association, 1984.

Index